How Covid Forever Changed Healthcare

Alexander Ruche, MSN, RN

Copyright © 2024 by Alexander Ruche, MSN,RN

All rights reserved.

No portion of this book may be reproduced in any form without written permission from the publisher or author, except as permitted by U.S. copyright law.

Contents

1. The Frontlines Redefined — 1
2. Public Health and Policy — 15
3. Technology and Innovation — 29
4. Patient Experience and Engagement — 43
5. Global Health Dynamics — 57
6. Mental Health and Resilience — 71
7. Ethical Considerations — 85
8. The Future of Healthcare Post-Covid — 102

Chapter One

The Frontlines Redefined

Nurses as Decision Makers

As the sun's first rays peeked through the half-drawn blinds of the bustling Intensive Medical Care Unit (IMCU), the air was electric with a mix of tension and determination. Here, in the heart of a metropolitan hospital, a revolution in healthcare was quietly taking place. It was a subtle transformation, yet its impact would reverberate through the very core of patient care.

At the center of this evolution were the nurses—my colleagues and I—no longer merely executors of doctors' orders but emerging as pivotal decision-makers in our own right. We had been thrust into the spotlight by a crisis that demanded rapid, on-the-ground decision-making, the likes of which we had never faced before.

The challenge was unprecedented: a novel virus that spread like wildfire, leaving us grappling with protocols that changed daily, if not hourly. We were sailing in uncharted waters, navigating by our wits and our intimate knowledge of patient care, honed by years of experience but tested by sheer necessity.

Our approach was both adaptive and innovative. Leveraging our frontline perspective, we began to implement immediate changes to care protocols that would normally have taken weeks of committee deliberations. We established new lines of communication with multidisciplinary teams, ensuring that our insights formed the backbone of patient care strategies.

The results were palpable. Patient outcomes improved as we shortened response times and tailored treatments more closely to individual needs. We became the eyes and ears of the healthcare team, our observations directly influencing the course of treatment in real-time.

Reflecting on those days, it's clear now that the crucible of the pandemic forged a new breed of nurse—the empowered practitioner. Yet, this evolution was not without its criticisms. Some viewed the shift towards nurse autonomy with skepticism, questioning whether the traditional hierarchies in healthcare were being disrupted too rapidly.

Visual aids, such as flowcharts of our newly implemented decision-making processes, adorned the walls of our break rooms and nursing stations, serving as a testament to our evolving roles. They were more than just diagrams; they represented a seismic shift in our professional identities.

This transformation extended far beyond the IMCU where I served. It was symptomatic of a larger narrative unfolding across the healthcare landscape. The pandemic had exposed the vulnerabilities of rigid hierarchies and the need for agile, informed decision-making at the point of care.

But what does this mean for the future of nursing? Have we reached a point of no return, where the traditional roles and expectations of nurses are forever altered?

Imagine, for a moment, a healthcare system where nurses regularly lead rounds, where their assessments carry as much weight as those of a physician. Is this the legacy of COVID-19, a reimagining of the nursing profession?

The questions linger, inviting contemplation. Yet, one thing is certain: the story of nursing in the post-COVID era is still being written, and the pen is now firmly in our hands.

As we close this chapter and look towards the horizon, we must ask ourselves: Are we ready to embrace the full scope of our potential, to step into the roles that circumstance has carved out for us? The answer lies not in the pages of history but in the actions, we take today and the choices we make for tomorrow.

Telehealth's Rapid Ascent

In the wake of the pandemic's tumultuous waves, another significant transformation was taking shape, reshaping the fabric of healthcare delivery. A quiet yet profound revolution was emerging from the shadows of necessity, paving the way for a future where face-to-face interactions between patient and provider were no longer the default setting. This was the meteoric rise of telehealth—a term once on the periphery of healthcare discussions, now thrust into the limelight as a cornerstone of medical practice.

Before the world was acquainted with the term 'COVID-19', telehealth was like a painting admired by a few for its potential yet left hanging in a seldom-visited gallery corner. Its earliest origins are traced back to the late 1950s and early 1960s, where it began as a modest endeavor by a few pioneering healthcare systems and academic medical centers. They utilized the technology of the time—closed-circuit televisions—to provide healthcare services over a distance. This was a time of experimentation and cautious exploration, limited by the technology available and overshadowed by the traditional in-person care model.

As the internet era dawned and technology evolved, telehealth began to paint its canvas with broader strokes. The major milestones in its journey map the integration of digital communications and information technologies in healthcare. These include the advent of high-speed internet, the proliferation of personal computers, and later, the ubiquity of smartphones. Each technological leap expanded telehealth's capabilities and reach, yet widespread adoption remained elusive. The potential was there, simmering beneath the surface, waiting for a catalyst to ignite its transformative power.

Pictures of early telehealth setups, showcasing clunky hardware and grainy video feeds, now serve as historical markers of how far we have come. Juxtapose these images with today's sleek telemedicine platforms, and one appreciates the remarkable evolution that has occurred.

One cannot discuss the ascent of telehealth without considering its impact on rural healthcare. For decades, individuals in remote locations grappled with the challenges of accessing timely and quality medical care. Geographic isolation, scarcity of specialists, and limited healthcare resources were barriers that made comprehensive care a distant dream for many. Here, telehealth began to show its true colors, bridging distances and bringing medical expertise to the doorsteps of those who might have otherwise gone without.

The variations in telehealth's evolution across different regions and cultures are notable. While some countries rapidly integrated telehealth services as a complement to traditional healthcare delivery, others faced infrastructural and regulatory hurdles that slowed its progress. However, the narrative remained consistent: telehealth was a key to unlocking better healthcare access, regardless of one's postal code.

The onset of the COVID-19 pandemic marked a turning point for telehealth, a moment where the world collectively turned its eyes towards this digital health service. Lockdowns and social distancing mandates necessitated a swift pivot from in-person consultations to virtual ones. Health systems and providers rapidly adapted, and patients, many experiencing telehealth for the first time, embraced its convenience and safety. Virtual consultations, once a fringe option, became the new norm in a matter of weeks.

But what are the modern interpretations of this digital consultation phenomenon? Today, telehealth is not merely a stopgap measure but an integral part of healthcare delivery. It has expanded beyond simple consultations to include remote monitoring, tele mental health, and mobile health applications. Technology has matured, enabling seamless interactions that rival, and sometimes surpass, the traditional office visit in effectiveness and efficiency.

This ascent has not been without its challenges and controversies. Questions of digital literacy, privacy concerns, and the nuances of patient-provider rapport in a virtual space have sparked discussions. Reimbursement policies and cross-state licensure laws for telehealth services continue to be points of contention, requiring ongoing policy innovation and adaptation.

Consider the profound impact telehealth has had on the rural landscape. Has it not transformed the very notion of accessibility in healthcare? Can we envision a future where rural patients no longer face the daunting prospect of long-distance travel for specialist consultations?

The truth is telehealth's rapid ascent is a testament to human ingenuity and adaptability in the face of crisis. It has permanently altered the healthcare terrain, opening doors to a future where quality care is not just a privilege of a few but a standard accessible to all.

As we reflect on this journey, we must ask ourselves: How will we continue to mold this digital frontier to meet the evolving needs of patients and providers alike? The answers will shape the narrative of healthcare for generations to come. For indeed, the ascent of telehealth is not just a tale of technology, but a story of resilience, innovation, and the enduring quest for a more equitable healthcare system.

The Evolution of Triage

In the labyrinth of healthcare evolution spurred by the Covid-19 pandemic, the life-or-death decisions made in the frenzied corridors of emergency rooms took on a new level of complexity. Triage, an age-old medical practice, was thrust into the harsh light of a global health crisis, revealing both its strengths and its vulnerabilities. As the world grappled with a virus that spared no nation, the necessity to adopt triage protocols became a matter of utmost urgency.

Imagine the scene: hospitals overrun, healthcare workers stretched to their limits, and resources dwindling. The pandemic underscored a stark reality – the existing triage systems were not fully equipped to handle the deluge of patients needing urgent care. A dilemma of epic proportions faced the medical community: how to prioritize care when the demand overwhelmingly exceeded the supply?

The consequences of inaction or misguided action were dire. Misallocation of limited resources could lead to increased mortality rates, healthcare worker burnout, and a loss of public trust in the health system. What then could be done to avert such an outcome?

A multifaceted solution began to take shape, rooted deeply in clinical pragmatism and ethical consideration. It involved revising triage protocols to be more dynamic, incorporating real-time data and predictive analytics. These revised protocols aimed to prioritize patients based not only on the immediacy of their condition but also on their likelihood of benefitting from treatment.

To implement these changes, a stepwise approach was undertaken. First, emergency departments were restructured to include Covid-19 specific zones, separating those with the virus from other patients, thus minimizing cross-infection. Next, triage teams were bolstered with additional training and support, emphasizing the importance of mental resilience in the face of overwhelming caseloads.

Technology played a pivotal role. Triage algorithms, once largely reliant on human judgment, began to integrate artificial intelligence to enhance decision-making. These AI systems were trained with vast datasets, learning to predict patient outcomes with a degree of accuracy that was once the sole domain of experienced clinicians.

The outcomes of these changes were notable. Hospitals that adopted the new triage systems reported more efficient use of intensive care units and ventilators, and a decrease in the time patients spent waiting for critical care. However, the transformation was not without its critics. Some questioned the ethical implications of algorithms making life-or-death decisions, igniting debates that would shape the future of medical ethics.

Could there have been an alternative to this approach? Certainly, some argued for a more conservative adjustment to triage, one that clung more closely to traditional methods. Yet, the unprecedented scale of the pandemic called for innovation – and fast. As such, while alternative solutions were considered, the urgency of the situation demanded swift, decisive action.

The pandemic, like a brutal teacher, imparted lessons that will reverberate through the halls of medicine for decades. It taught us that triage, a system as old as medicine itself, must evolve to meet the challenges of an ever-changing world of threats. As healthcare providers continue to navigate the post-pandemic landscape, they do so with a renewed understanding of triage's critical role in saving lives.

The question now lingers in the air, heavy with the weight of responsibility: How will we apply these hard-earned lessons to future crises? Will we allow ourselves to be caught unprepared again, or will we take the necessary steps to ensure that our triage systems are as resilient as the healthcare workers who operate them?

As the chapters of this pandemic close and new ones begin, the story of triage's evolution remains a testament to humanity's capacity to adapt and overcome. It is a narrative not just of survival but of our collective resolve to emerge from crisis with a stronger, more equitable healthcare system for all.

Cross-Training for Flexibility

In the wake of the pandemic's tumultuous upheaval, the healthcare industry found itself navigating uncharted waters. The virus, like a storm, left no shore untouched, altering the landscape of medical practice with a force that called for swift adaptation and reformation. Notably, the concept of cross-training staff emerged as a lighthouse in the tempest, guiding healthcare facilities toward a more agile and resilient future.

As we delve into the heart of this transformation, let us consider the profound impact of cross-training on the healthcare workforce.

Picture a hospital where nurses, traditionally specialized in specific areas, are now adept in multiple disciplines, moving fluidly between departments as the tides of patient needs rise and fall. This is not just a hypothetical scenario but a burgeoning reality in the post-Covid era.

The proposition is clear: by cross-training staff, healthcare systems can cultivate a workforce versatile enough to respond to dynamically changing needs. This claim rests on the bedrock of recent experience, where the sudden influx of patients necessitated a rapid reconfiguration of roles and responsibilities.

Take, for instance, the evidence presented by a large metropolitan hospital. In the throes of the pandemic's peak, they initiated a cross-training program for their staff. Nurses from elective surgery units, which saw a dramatic decrease in activity, were retrained to support the intensive care and emergency departments, which were buckling under the strain of Covid-19 cases. The program's success was not merely anecdotal; patient outcomes improved, wait times decreased, and the hospital's overall capacity to respond to the crisis was markedly enhanced.

Yet, to appreciate these benefits fully, one must scrutinize the underlying details. Cross-training enabled a more efficient allocation of human resources, as staff could be deployed where they were most needed at any given moment. It also fostered a deeper sense of camaraderie and mutual understanding among different departments, breaking down silos that had previously hindered collaboration.

However, this narrative is not devoid of counterarguments. Skeptics point to the potential for diluted expertise and the risk of overwhelming healthcare workers with the demands of multiple roles. Surely, there is validity in cautioning against a one-size-fits-all approach to staff deployment.

In response, it is essential to clarify that cross-training is not about creating jack-of-all-trades practitioners but rather about equipping staff with additional skills to enhance their core competencies. Programs are carefully designed to ensure that while flexibility is achieved, the depth of knowledge in each practitioner's primary area of expertise is not compromised.

Moreover, the argument for cross-training extends beyond immediate crisis response. The healthcare landscape is ever evolving, and with the emergence of new diseases, treatments, and technologies, a flexible workforce is better positioned to adapt and thrive. Evidence of this can be seen in the continued professional development of staff who, empowered by their expanded skill sets, are contributing to innovations in patient care and operational efficiency.

As we draw this examination to a close, the assertion that cross-training is a necessity in modern healthcare stands reinforced. The pandemic has irrevocably shifted the paradigm, and in this new reality, the ability of healthcare systems to remain flexible and responsive is paramount.

We are left to ponder, then, what the future holds for healthcare delivery. Will cross-training become the new standard, a staple in curricula and hospital protocols alike? As we chart the course forward, one truth remains evident: the lessons learned during the pandemic have laid the foundation for a more resilient, adaptable, and unified healthcare workforce.

In the final analysis, the narrative of healthcare's transformation is still being written. But if the chapters of the pandemic have taught us anything, it is that flexibility is not just a strategy but a survival imperative. Cross-training, as a manifestation of this flexibility, has proven itself a beacon of hope and a catalyst for change in the enduring mission to safeguard human health.

Mental Health of Healthcare Workers

In the crucible of the Covid-19 pandemic, the world bore witness to the extraordinary resilience and dedication of healthcare workers. Yet amidst the applause and accolades, a silent struggle unfolded behind the scenes—a toll on mental health that would leave indelible scars on those at the frontlines. This chapter seeks to illuminate the psychological repercussions of the pandemic on healthcare professionals and to chart a course for healing and support.

The importance of addressing the mental well-being of our healthcare workers cannot be overstated. As we proceed, we will explore a list of critical points concerning their mental health, each accompanied by a deeper analysis, real-world evidence, and practical applications for ongoing support.

Increased Risk of Burnout
Psychological Trauma and PTSD
Elevated Rates of Anxiety and Depression
Strategies for Institutional Support
Coping Mechanisms and Self-Care
Increased Risk of Burnout

The specter of burnout among healthcare workers has long haunted medical institutions, but the pandemic magnified this risk to unprecedented levels. Burnout, characterized by emotional exhaustion, depersonalization, and a diminished sense of personal accomplishment, became a common refrain for those laboring under the relentless pressure of Covid care.

Evidence of this escalation is found in numerous studies, including one survey where nearly half of the healthcare workers reported symptoms consistent with burnout. Testimonials from doctors and nurses recount endless shifts, grueling decision-making, and the emotional toll of high patient mortality—factors which contributed to this mental fatigue.

In terms of practical applications, hospitals and clinics have begun implementing strategies to mitigate burnout, such as offering mental health days, providing on-site counseling services, and ensuring reasonable work hours when possible. These measures are crucial, not only for the well-being of the staff but also for the quality of patient care they can provide.

Psychological Trauma and PTSD

Healthcare workers, thrust onto the frontlines, often bore witness to harrowing scenes that could inflict lasting psychological trauma. The relentless wave of critically ill patients, coupled with the fear of contagion and the heartbreak of isolated patients dying without family, planted the seeds for post-traumatic stress disorder (PTSD).

The narrative is supported by research highlighting the prevalence of PTSD symptoms among healthcare professionals during and after the Covid-19 surges. Personal stories shared by emergency room personnel reveal the nightmares and flashbacks that haunt them, a testament to the war-like conditions they endured.

To combat this, institutions have established peer support programs and trauma-informed care training, equipping staff with tools to recognize and address PTSD. Additionally, creating spaces for healthcare workers to share their experiences has fostered community and collective healing.

Elevated Rates of Anxiety and Depression

Amidst the uncertainty of the pandemic's progression, healthcare workers grappled with heightened levels of anxiety and depression. The constant concern over personal safety, the wellbeing of their families, and the emotional burden of patient care amplified these mental health challenges.

Quantitative data underscores the spike in reported cases of anxiety and depression among medical staff, with certain studies indicating that one in three healthcare workers experienced symptoms during the pandemic. The personal accounts of clinicians and support staff lay bare the psychological toll of living in a state of high alert for months on end.

In response, many healthcare systems have expanded access to mental health resources, including hotlines, virtual therapy sessions, and resilience-building workshops. These initiatives aim to provide a lifeline to those struggling and to normalize the conversation around mental health.

Strategies for Institutional Support

Institutional support emerged as a cornerstone for addressing the mental health crisis within healthcare. Recognizing the necessity for systemic change, healthcare institutions began reevaluating and restructuring their approach to employee wellness.

Success stories from various hospitals illustrate the implementation of comprehensive support systems, which include proactive mental health screenings, the introduction of wellness programs, and the appointment of chief wellness officers dedicated to staff mental health.

Coping Mechanisms and Self-Care

The personal responsibility of healthcare workers in managing their mental health gained renewed focus. Self-care, once an afterthought in the demanding healthcare environment, took center stage as a vital component of professional sustainability.

Narratives of healthcare workers finding solace in meditation, exercise, and artistic expression have proliferated, underscoring the diverse ways individuals cope with stress. Moreover, the sharing of these experiences has encouraged a culture where self-care is not only accepted but actively promoted.

As we bridge the gap between the harrowing experiences of the past and the hope for a more supportive future, it becomes clear that the mental health of healthcare workers is not merely a personal concern but a collective responsibility. The strategies and support systems discussed herein represent a starting point, but the journey to comprehensive mental wellness for our healthcare heroes is ongoing and must be pursued with unwavering commitment.

As we contemplate the gravity of the pandemic's impact, one cannot help but ask: are we doing enough to support the mental health of those who care for us? The answer lies not in the silence of reticence but in the actions we take to ensure no healthcare worker has to suffer in silence. Through empathy, understanding, and tangible support, we can begin to repay the incalculable debt we owe to those who stood between us and the abyss.

Chapter Two

Public Health and Policy

Pandemic Preparedness

In the shadow of a world reshaped by Covid-19, the term "pandemic preparedness" has been etched into the collective consciousness like a scar from a wound that has only just begun to heal. It speaks of vigilance, of lessons hard learned, and of a future that demands our foresight. But to navigate the intricacies of this new terrain, one must first grasp the lexicon that defines it.

Pandemic preparedness, public health infrastructure, zoonotic transmission, health equity, telehealth, and infection control—these are not merely terms to be memorized; they are concepts to be understood. They embody the collective knowledge gleaned from our recent trials and the strategies to be employed for the safeguarding of tomorrow.

Pandemic preparedness is the strategic approach to ensuring that systems are in place to detect, respond to, and prevent the spread of infectious diseases on a global scale. It encompasses the stockpiling of essential medical supplies, development of rapid testing procedures, and establishment of protocols for swift vaccine production.

Public health infrastructure is the framework upon which the well-being of a population is built. It includes hospitals, laboratories, workforce, data systems, and the legislative policies that govern them. This infrastructure becomes the frontline defense in the face of an emerging health crisis.

Zoonotic transmission, a term that has garnered much attention in recent times, refers to the passage of pathogens from animals to humans. Understanding this process is key to pre-empting outbreaks, as many of the deadliest viruses known to humanity—including Covid-19—have their origins in wildlife.

Health equity is the pursuit of eliminating disparities in health outcomes and access to care across different demographics, ensuring that every individual has a fair opportunity to achieve their full health potential regardless of social position or other socially determined circumstances.

Telehealth, once a peripheral option, has been thrust into the limelight, offering medical consultations and care through digital platforms. This innovation in healthcare delivery has proven essential in reducing physical contact during the pandemic while maintaining continuous access to medical services.

Infection control is a set of practices employed to minimize the spread of infectious diseases. These include hand hygiene, use of personal protective equipment (PPE), and isolation protocols. The effectiveness of these practices has been highlighted by the pandemic's challenges.

Each term unfolds into a narrative, weaving into the fabric of reality. Pandemic preparedness is not an abstract concept but a tangible action, reflected in the stockpiles of masks and vaccines. Public health infrastructure is visible in the hospital wards and the tireless professionals who staff them. Zoonotic transmission brings to mind the images of wildlife markets and the sobering realization of our interconnectedness with nature.

Health equity casts a spotlight on the map, revealing the stark contrasts between affluent neighborhoods and underserved communities, while telehealth bridges distances, bringing the physician's expertise into the quiet privacy of a patient's home. Infection control takes shape in the ubiquitous bottles of hand sanitizer and the signs that remind us to keep our distance.

One must pause and consider—what do these terms mean in the scope of our daily lives? How have our routines been altered by the newfound necessity of infection control? Can we envision a future where health equity is not an aspiration but a reality? And as we lean on the crutch of telehealth, do we not marvel at the resilience of human innovation?

In the silence of a one-line paragraph, a truth resounds: the pandemic has ended, but its lessons endure.

Vivid imagery paints the new dawn of healthcare, where the air in a hospital room is filtered with a vigilance born of recent memory, and the once-empty halls now echo with the footsteps of those who have come to trust in the robustness of reimagined public health strategies.

Consider the healthcare worker, donning their PPE with the precision of a ritual, their movements a dance of muscle memory and responsibility. Imagine the screens ablaze with the faces of patients and doctors, telehealth consultations unfolding with the ease of a conversation across the dinner table.

Amidst the rhythm of these transformations, quotations from frontline workers resonate, echoing their experiences: "We adapted because we had to, and in doing so, we rewrote the playbook on healthcare delivery," confides a nurse, her eyes reflecting both the fatigue and the resolve etched by the pandemic.

In the unfolding of this narrative, the story is not told; it is shown. The reader does not simply learn of the gaps in public health infrastructure—they see the lines at the testing centers, the disparities in vaccine distribution, the ingenuity of makeshift clinics. They witness the bending, but not breaking, of systems and spirits.

As the chapter closes, the page remains open, not with a question, but with an invitation to ponder, to engage, to remember. For in the chronicles of pandemic preparedness, the tale is ongoing, and the ink is still wet upon the legacy of how Covid changed healthcare forever.

Vaccine Rollout Strategies

The vaccine rollout has become a defining chapter in the saga of the Covid-19 pandemic, a multifaceted narrative of triumphs and tribulations that has seen nations grappling with unprecedented challenges. Across continents, the strategies employed to distribute vaccines have varied widely, each with its own set of outcomes that demand a closer examination. The significance of these approaches cannot be overstated, for they hold the key to unlocking the resilience of our healthcare systems in the face of future crises.

The purpose of this analysis is to dissect the global tapestry of vaccine distribution strategies to not only illuminate their effectiveness but also to glean lessons for the future. As we delve into this inquiry, we shall establish criteria based on factors such as speed of distribution, equity of access, and impact on public health outcomes, setting a stage for a thorough and balanced comparison.

Let us begin with the similarities that have emerged in this global endeavor. Many countries prioritized healthcare workers and the elderly in the early phases, recognizing their vulnerability and essential roles. Mass vaccination sites and innovative drive-through services became a common sight, aiming to inoculate large numbers swiftly. The spirit of urgency was universal, a shared heartbeat driving the campaign against the relentless virus.

Yet, as we pivot to the contrasts, the nuances of each strategy take shape. In countries like Israel and the United Kingdom, centralized public health systems allowed for more streamlined and coordinated efforts, resulting in higher vaccination rates in the initial months. Contrast this with the United States, where a decentralized approach with federal guidance led to a patchwork of strategies, varying from state to state, often mired in complexity.

Visual aids, such as comparative graphs and maps, delineate these stark differences, illustrating the disparate speeds of vaccine deployment and the consequent curves of infection rates and mortality. The images serve as silent witnesses to the successes and the shortcomings, guiding the reader's eye through the labyrinth of data.

The analysis reveals a tale of two worlds—one where access to vaccines was swift and equitable, and another where scarcity and inequity cast long shadows. In wealthy nations, surplus vaccines and robust infrastructure paved the way for a quicker return to semblance of normalcy. Meanwhile, countries with limited resources faced delayed vaccine deliveries and logistical challenges that hampered their response.

What do these comparisons tell us? They speak of a broader implication: the intrinsic link between healthcare infrastructure and pandemic resilience. The stark disparities in vaccine rollout have underscored the need for a global framework that ensures equitable access to life-saving vaccines for all nations, rich or poor.

Can the reader not help but ponder the contemporary relevance of these insights? As new variants emerge and the threat of future pandemics looms, the question arises: how can we fortify our collective defenses? The answer lies partly in the lessons learned from the strategies we have scrutinized.

As we reflect on the profound impact of vaccine distribution approaches, we encounter the stories of individuals: a nurse in a remote clinic, finally receiving her dose after months of anxious waiting; a grandparent embracing their grandchild, the simple act made possible by a jab in the arm. Their narratives are the threads woven into the larger fabric of our shared human experience.

Does the image not resonate—a bustling vaccination center, the air punctuated with the soft hum of efficiency, as one by one, individuals reclaim a piece of their pre-pandemic lives? It is here, in the rhythm of these personal victories, that we find a cadence of hope, a testament to humanity's collective endeavor.

In conclusion, the vaccine rollout strategies have painted a complex mosaic of human ingenuity and perseverance. As we stand on the threshold of a post-pandemic era, we must carry forward the wisdom gleaned from this pivotal moment in history. Let us forge ahead, not with a sense of finality, but with the knowledge that our actions today will shape the healthcare landscape of tomorrow.

The Role of Government in Healthcare

In the long shadow of human history, the arrival of the novel coronavirus marked a turning point. A global health crisis of a magnitude unseen in over a century, Covid-19 was a specter that swept across continents, sparing no nation in its path. As countries scrambled to respond, it became increasingly clear that the role of government would be pivotal in shaping the trajectory of the pandemic and, subsequently, the future of healthcare.

Travel back in time to the early days of the outbreak—Wuhan, late 2019. A mysterious illness emerges, one that would soon reveal itself to be a harbinger of upheaval. From those initial whispers of a novel virus, the world watched with bated breath as the situation quickly escalated into a global emergency. Governments were thrust into the spotlight, with each decision and action (or lack thereof) under the microscope of an anxious global populace.

Historical milestones in public health, such as the Spanish Flu of 1918 and the more recent H1N1 influenza pandemic, provided some roadmap for nations. Yet, Covid-19 presented unique challenges that demanded innovative responses. Governments around the world took on various roles—patron, regulator, coordinator, and provider—to steer their nations through the storm.

From past to present, we see the evolution of government intervention in healthcare. The pandemic accelerated the adoption of telemedicine, spurred the rapid development of vaccines, and catalyzed a reevaluation of public health preparedness and healthcare delivery systems. It compelled governments to act with unprecedented speed and scale, often in collaboration with private sectors and international bodies.

Why does history matter now, in the context of a modern healthcare crisis? Understanding the successes and failures of the past allows us to refine our approach to current and future challenges. It highlights the need for robust, adaptable systems and for governance that can quickly mobilize resources and enact effective policies.

As we segue into the story of government intervention during the Covid-19 pandemic, let us delve into the details of this complex narrative. What strategies did governments employ to mitigate the spread of the virus? How did they secure and distribute the precious cargo of vaccines? What role did international cooperation play in bridging the gap between nations of varying wealth and resources?

In the depths of the crisis, governments around the world faced a daunting task: to protect public health while managing the economic and social fallout. Some took aggressive measures, implementing strict lockdowns and travel bans. Others adopted a more laissez-faire approach, attempting to balance economic pressures with public health concerns. The outcomes were as diverse as the strategies themselves, painting a picture of a world grappling with an invisible, yet omnipotent enemy.

How did these varied approaches impact the course of the pandemic, and what can they tell us about the role of government in managing a healthcare crisis? Can we discern patterns of success that might guide future policy decisions?

Consider the case of South Korea, which employed a rigorous system of testing, contact tracing, and isolation, harnessing technology and a centralized healthcare system to remarkable effect. Contrast this with Brazil, where conflicting messages and political divisions led to a disjointed response, with devastating consequences.

The narrative of government intervention is not just a tale of strategies and systems—it is also a human story. It is the story of frontline workers, toiling tirelessly in hospitals stretched to their limits. It is the tale of community leaders, stepping up to fill voids left by national policies, and of ordinary citizens, navigating the new realities of lockdowns and social distancing.

HOW COVID FOREVER CHANGED HEALTHCARE

What lessons does this pandemic hold for the role of government in healthcare? As we emerge from the acute phase of the crisis, the importance of preparedness, agility, and equity in healthcare is more evident than ever. Governments must take these lessons to heart, building systems that can not only withstand future pandemics but also address the everyday health needs of their populations.

In the aftermath of Covid-19, the role of government in healthcare has been irrevocably altered. The pandemic has laid bare the vulnerabilities in our global health systems and highlighted the critical need for effective governance. As we look ahead, the question looms large: how will governments adapt to ensure a healthier, more resilient future for all?

The transformation of healthcare, catalyzed by the trials of Covid-19, offers both a cautionary tale and a beacon of hope. As we turn the page on this chapter of history, it is incumbent upon us all—policymakers, healthcare professionals, and citizens—to reflect on the lessons learned and to forge a path forward that is informed by the past, responsive to the present, and anticipatory of the future.

And so, dear reader, as you digest the gravity of the role that government has played in shaping healthcare amidst a pandemic, do you not find yourself pondering the road ahead? Does the thought not stir within you, a resolve to advocate for a system that is not merely reactive, but proactively fortified against the unknown perils that lie in wait?

We stand now at a crossroads, with the power to reimagine the future of healthcare. Let us proceed with wisdom, compassion, and the collective will to create a world that is healthier, more equitable, and better prepared for the challenges to come.

Healthcare Access in Crisis

The core of the crisis remains glaringly exposed: access to healthcare during a pandemic. The novel coronavirus unveiled the stark disparities and inefficiencies within our healthcare systems, highlighting a problem that resonates deeply with anyone who has ever sought medical care in such tumultuous times. But what exactly is the nature of this access conundrum that our society faces?

Imagine a world where the zip code of your birth determines your health destiny, where invisible lines divide not just neighborhoods but also life expectancies. Covid-19 exacerbated this divide, laying bare the inequities that pervade healthcare access. The virus did not discriminate, but our systems did, resulting in vastly different outcomes for the wealthy and the impoverished, for the urban dweller and the rural inhabitant.

Can you visualize the long queues for testing, the desperate scramble for hospital beds, the palpable fear in the eyes of the underinsured? This was the grim reality for many, particularly those in marginalized communities. The pandemic became a magnifying glass, revealing the grim tapestry of a healthcare system fraught with disparities.

Let me share with you the story of Maria, a single mother of three in a densely populated city. Maria worked two jobs to keep her family afloat and lacked health insurance. When the virus claimed her neighborhood, her fear was twofold: the threat of the disease and the potential financial ruin from seeking care. Maria's tale is but one thread in a sprawling narrative of struggle that so many have endured.

The stakes? They could not be higher. The cost of inaction is measured in human lives. Each day without equitable healthcare access means more people like Maria face impossible choices. The urgency to act, to reform, to innovate cannot be overstated. The pandemic has not just been a health crisis—it's been a clarion call for change.

But where do we go from here? Your journey through these pages will not only confront the harsh realities but also illuminate the path forward. Innovative solutions have emerged from the crucible of this pandemic—telehealth services have burgeoned, virtual care has become the new frontline, and community health initiatives have taken a pronounced role in reaching the underserved.

Dive deep with me into the fabric of these innovations. Picture a future where telehealth consultations bridge the gap between rural and urban care. Envision mobile health clinics winding their way through underserved neighborhoods, bringing hope and healing. These are not mere daydreams; they are real, tangible advancements that have sprung from necessity and are reshaping the landscape of healthcare.

But how can this be sustained? How do we ensure these innovations are not merely a flash in the pan but a durable part of a reformed healthcare system? The answers lie in policy, in investment, and in a societal commitment to healthcare as a fundamental right, not a privilege.

Consider the ripple effects of a well-accessed healthcare system: a healthier workforce, a reduced burden on emergency services, and ultimately, a stronger, more resilient population. The benefits are manifold, the impact multi-generational.

You might ask, "What can I, as an individual, contribute to this monumental task?" The answer is both simple and profound: your voice, your advocacy, and your informed choices can steer the tide toward a more equitable healthcare future.

As you delve further into the ensuing chapters, you will encounter stories of resilience and innovation, of communities banding together to fill the voids left by inadequate systems. You will learn of policies that have the potential to reshape access to healthcare—not as a commodity, but as an inalienable right.

We stand at the precipice of a new era in healthcare. The pandemic has been a crucible, one that has forged new tools and strategies, but it has also revealed the fractures that run deep in our systems. It is incumbent upon us to wield these tools with wisdom and to mend the fractures with a resolve that is unyielding.

And so, as you absorb the gravity of what has transpired and the promise of what may come, I invite you to join in the dialogue, to challenge the status quo, and to envision a world where healthcare access in crisis is not a tale of woe but a narrative of triumph over adversity. For it is only through collective will and concerted effort that we can hope to write the next chapter—one where healthcare has changed, not just for the duration of a pandemic, but forever.

Data Transparency and Public Trust

In a world where the invisible enemy, a virus, wreaked havoc on the very fabric of our society, transparency and trust emerged as the twin pillars of an effective public health response. How did we arrive at a juncture where these two elements became so crucial? And what roadmap can we follow to ensure they remain at the forefront of any future health crisis management?

Understanding the significance of data transparency is akin to recognizing the need for a compass during a storm. It guides us, offering a beacon of truth in a sea of uncertainty. The goal here is clear: to establish a health care system where data is not only accurate but readily accessible, ensuring that every decision, from policymaking to personal health choices, is informed and trustworthy.

To achieve this, several prerequisites must be firmly in place. A robust technological infrastructure that can handle vast amounts of data is non-negotiable. Equally important is the establishment of stringent data governance policies that protect privacy while promoting sharing. Healthcare professionals must be trained in data literacy, and the public educated on the importance of data in health outcomes.

Picture a broad canvas, painted with the broad strokes of policy, technology, and education. This is the overview of our journey towards data transparency and public trust. The details in this canvas reveal a meticulous process, each brushstroke representing a deliberate action towards our goal.

Delving into the details, we first encounter the challenge of collecting accurate data. This involves setting up widespread testing centers, ensuring laboratory capacity, and establishing reporting protocols that are both timely and verifiable. The process continues with the dissemination of this data, which requires sophisticated yet user-friendly platforms that allow the public to access real-time information.

Imagine a dashboard where you can track the spread of a virus in your community, know the capacity of local hospitals, and understand the efficacy of implemented health measures. It's not the stuff of imagination; such systems have been developed and deployed, albeit with varying degrees of success.

But what happens when the data conflicts with the narrative, or worse, is used to propagate misinformation? Herein lies the importance of our tips and warnings. Transparency is not just about making data available; it's about presenting it in a context that is understandable and actionable. It demands a careful balance: too little information breeds suspicion, while too much can cause confusion.

How do we verify that our pursuit of transparency is yielding the desired trust? Surveys and feedback mechanisms are key tools that gauge public sentiment. Trust, after all, is not a static entity but a dynamic relationship that must be nurtured and measured.

It is, however, inevitable that challenges will arise. Misinterpretation of data, technical glitches, and resistance to change are but a few obstacles on this path. Troubleshooting these issues requires a proactive stance, ready to address concerns, correct errors, and adapt strategies in real-time.

Let's consider a scenario where a data breach occurs. Immediate action must be taken to secure the system, followed by transparent communication with the public about what happened, how it was resolved, and what measures are being implemented to prevent future breaches. This open approach builds trust even in the face of adversity.

As we navigate the intricacies of this journey, we must not forget the power of stories. Recall the healthcare professionals who tirelessly collected and reported data, often at great personal risk. Envision the community leaders who used this data to make informed decisions, guiding their neighborhoods with wisdom and foresight.

Now, pause for a moment. Have you ever questioned the source of the health statistics you read? Have you considered how they were gathered, who verified them, and what they truly mean for you and your loved ones? It's in asking these questions that we begin to appreciate the importance of transparency and public trust.

We stand at a crossroads, armed with the knowledge that data transparency is not merely a technical endeavor but a covenant with the public—a promise of honesty, clarity, and respect. As the pages of this book unfold, so too should our commitment to a healthcare system that values and upholds these principles. For it is only through this unwavering dedication to transparency and trust that we can hope to face any future health crises with the unity and resilience that our global community so desperately needs.

Chapter Three

Technology and Innovation

AI in Diagnosis and Treatment

In the wake of a global pandemic, the landscape of healthcare has been irrevocably altered, opening new vistas where technology and medicine converge. Chief among the harbingers of this transformation is artificial intelligence (AI), a beacon of hope in a sea of data, illuminating paths to diagnoses and treatments once shrouded in the shadow of uncertainty.

Imagine a world where the vast compendium of medical knowledge is distilled into a form that is not only accessible but also actionable within moments. This is the promise of AI in healthcare—a promise that is already being fulfilled in clinics and hospitals around the world.

At the heart of AI's revolutionary impact is its unparalleled ability to manage and interpret patient data. Every symptom, test result, and medical image represents a piece of the puzzle that AI can piece together with astonishing speed and accuracy. By harnessing the power of algorithms and machine learning, AI systems are trained to recognize patterns that may elude even the most experienced clinicians.

Consider the case of a patient with a rare condition that baffles local doctors. In the past, this might have meant a long and arduous journey through the healthcare system, fraught with uncertainty and delay. Today, AI can compare the patient's data against global databases, identifying potential diagnoses and suggesting treatment plans that have been effective for similar cases.

The power of AI is not limited to rare diseases. In the realm of cancer treatment, for example, AI algorithms analyze medical images to detect tumors with greater precision than ever before. These systems can even predict how different cancers will respond to various treatments, personalizing therapy to the individual's unique genetic makeup.

Yet, AI's role in healthcare is not without its critics. Some fear the depersonalization of medicine, where the warmth of human touch is supplanted by the cold efficiency of algorithms. Others raise concerns about privacy and the security of sensitive patient data in the hands of AI systems. These perspectives are important, reminding us that technology should enhance, not replace, the patient-caregiver relationship.

To appreciate the full scope of AI's impact, one must look at the numbers. Studies show that AI can reduce diagnostic errors, which account for a significant portion of medical complications. In some cases, the use of AI has led to a 50% reduction in false positives and false negatives, a statistic that translates to lives saved and improved.

While discussing these advancements, it's crucial to demystify the jargon that often accompanies conversations about AI. Terms like 'deep learning' and 'neural networks' can seem daunting, but at their core, they refer to the ability of computers to learn from data and improve over time, much like a human apprentice learning a trade.

As we draw the curtain on this exploration of AI in healthcare, let's crystallize the key takeaways: AI is reshaping the diagnosis and treatment of diseases by harnessing the power of patient data, improving outcomes through precision medicine, and challenging us to reconcile the benefits of technology with the timeless values of compassion and empathy. The road ahead is laden with potential, and as we march forward, we must do so with a careful balance between innovation and the human touch that lies at the heart of healing.

Wearable Health Monitors

The fabric of healthcare is woven with threads of innovation, each strand representing a breakthrough, a turning point, a moment of metamorphosis. Wearable health monitors are one such filament, a testimony to how personal tech can become an integral part of our wellness and medical care. Let us embark on a journey through time, tracing the origins and evolution of these devices, to understand how they are reshaping the landscape of healthcare in the wake of Covid-19.

In the early days, the concept of monitoring one's health was largely confined to the walls of a clinic or hospital. The inception of wearable health technology can be traced back to the humble pedometer, a simple device created in the 1960s, designed to encourage physical activity by counting steps. Yet, who could have foreseen the tremendous strides this field would take in the ensuing decades?

Fast forward to the 21st century, and the milestones are nothing short of remarkable. The major leaps began with heart rate monitors in the 1980s, initially bulky and unwieldy, evolving to sleek, wrist-worn devices by the 2000s. The advent of smartwatches and fitness trackers in the early 2010s marked a pivotal moment, as they began to furnish a wider array of biometric data at a glance.

Enhancing our understanding, one may visualize the transformation: diagrams of early pedometers beside modern smartwatches, images of first-generation heart rate straps juxtaposed with current, sensor-laden wearables. These visuals serve to underscore the rapid progression from simple to sophisticated.

Diversity blooms in the realm of technology, and wearable health monitors are no exception. Across cultures and regions, adaptation has varied. In some parts of the world, these devices quickly became fashionable accessories, while in others, they were adopted more cautiously, often by those with a pressing health need or interest in fitness.

In recent years, and especially since Covid-19 reshaped our world, the trajectory of wearable health monitors has skyrocketed. The race to monitor one's own health data has become not just a trend, but a necessity for many. From tracking oxygen saturation levels to detecting irregular heart rhythms, these gadgets are increasingly seen as potential lifesavers.

But it hasn't all been smooth sailing. Challenges and controversies have emerged alongside the technological triumphs. Questions regarding data privacy and security have sparked heated debates. How can we ensure that sensitive health information remains confidential and secure?

Moreover, there has been a turning point in the integration of wearables into patient care. Notably, during the pandemic, remote patient monitoring became essential, allowing healthcare providers to track patients' health without the need for physical interaction. This adaptation may have been born out of necessity, but it has opened doors to a new realm of possibilities for patient care.

HOW COVID FOREVER CHANGED HEALTHCARE

Have you ever paused to consider how these devices might continue to evolve? The modern interpretations of wearable health monitors are moving towards ever-more seamless integration into our lives. Think smart fabrics with embedded sensors or even temporary tattoos that monitor vitals. The future holds a vision where monitoring health could be as routine as checking the time on a watch.

Yet, as we marvel at these breakthroughs, one must remember the power of simplicity. The true essence of these devices lies not in their complexity but in their ability to provide clear, actionable insights into our health.

One must also give a nod to the rhythm and cadence of this evolution. It's a dance of technology and medicine, where each step forward is measured, deliberate, with the occasional bold leap into the unknown.

In the words of a pioneering researcher in the field, "Wearable health monitors represent the democratization of healthcare." These devices empower individuals to take charge of their own well-being, bridging the gap between patient and provider, and weaving a new narrative in the story of healthcare.

As we close this chapter, let us reflect. Wearable health monitors have come a long way from their rudimentary origins. Today, they stand as sentinels of health, guardians of our well-being. In a world forever altered by a pandemic, they are a testament to the resilience and ingenuity of the human spirit, a beacon of hope in our continuous quest for a healthier tomorrow.

Remote Patient Monitoring

In the stillness of a home, where the echoes of bustling clinics fade, the pulse of healthcare transformation beats strong. It is here, in the intimate corners of personal space, that the revolution of remote patient monitoring (RPM) is quietly rewriting the narrative of patient management. As the world grapples with the aftermath of a global pandemic, the practice of healthcare is undergoing a seismic shift, with RPM at its epicenter.

Imagine the plight of millions, confined to their homes, as a virulent virus lurks outside. A pressing need arises: How do we provide continuous care for those who are isolated, to the chronically ill who cannot risk exposure, to the elderly whose frailty makes every trip to the doctor a gamble? The issue at hand is clear—traditional healthcare models are not equipped for such widespread and sustained disruption.

Left unaddressed, the disconnect between patients and healthcare systems could lead to deteriorating health outcomes, increased hospital readmissions, and a greater burden on already overwhelmed medical facilities. The implications are dire, stretching beyond individual well-being to the health of communities at large.

But what if we could bridge this gap? What if technology could bring the watchful eyes of healthcare into our homes? This is not the fodder of science fiction; it is the pragmatic solution RPM presents. With RPM, patients can be monitored by healthcare professionals from a distance, using medical devices that relay information such as heart rate, blood pressure, blood sugar levels, and oxygen saturation in real time.

To implement RPM, a clear blueprint must be laid out. It begins with equipping patients with the necessary devices—sleek, user-friendly tools that seamlessly integrate into their daily lives. Next, secure and robust software platforms must be established to transmit data effectively and maintain patient privacy. Healthcare professionals are then trained to interpret this data, making informed decisions about patient care without the need for face-to-face interaction.

Evidence of RPM's efficacy is not merely anecdotal; it is supported by numbers and outcomes. Studies have shown that RPM can lead to significant reductions in hospital readmission rates, particularly for patients with chronic conditions. In a world where healthcare costs are skyrocketing, RPM stands as a beacon of efficiency, ensuring that resources are allocated judiciously, that patients receive the right care at the right time.

While RPM is a compelling solution, it is not the sole answer. Alternative approaches, such as telehealth consultations and mobile health apps, also offer valuable support to patient management. The merits of each option must be weighed, with a tailored approach that best suits the individual needs of each patient.

Consider the rhythm of a patient's day: the morning blood pressure check, the post-lunch glucose reading, the evening medication reminder. RPM becomes a harmonious part of this daily cadence, a silent partner in the quest for health. Stories emerge of lives transformed—of the heart failure patient who avoided emergency room visits, of the diabetic whose condition is now expertly managed from afar.

Is it not empowering to envision a future where healthcare transcends physical boundaries, where each patient is enfolded in a network of care that extends beyond the hospital room? This is the legacy of COVID-19, a chapter that, though marked by hardship, has catalyzed an evolution in patient care that will resonate for generations.

As we tread further into this era of modern healthcare, it is essential to remember the core tenet that guides our journey: the well-being of the patient. RPM is more than technology; it is a commitment to preserving human health with every beat, every breath, every blood sugar level monitored. It represents a collective stride towards a future where healthcare is not only reactive but proactive, where every individual is afforded the dignity of comprehensive care, regardless of circumstance.

In the quiet of the night, when the worries of health seem most profound, the reassuring hum of remote patient monitoring devices stands as a testament to the enduring spirit of innovation—a reminder that even in our most isolated moments, we are never truly alone in our quest for health and well-being.

The Growth of Health Apps

In the landscape of modern medicine, where innovation and technology are as essential as the stethoscope and the syringe, there lies a new frontier that beckons with the promise of empowerment and autonomy. Amidst this terrain, health apps emerge as the digital conduits connecting patients to a more personalized healthcare experience. They represent a pivotal shift in the dynamic of patient engagement and self-management, a shift amplified by the global sweep of a pandemic that has left indelible marks on the canvas of healthcare.

Dawn breaks with the soft glow of a smartphone screen, illuminating the contours of a new routine. With the tap of a finger, individuals greet the day not just with a clock's alarm but with a health app's reminder to take their medication, to hydrate, to prepare for a day attuned to their well-being. But is this digital intervention merely a convenience, or does it signal a deeper transformation in the way we manage our health?

The claim is clear: health apps have revolutionized patient engagement and self-management, fostering an environment where individuals are not passive recipients of healthcare but active participants in the maintenance of their well-being. This assertion, bold in its implications, is not without concrete evidence to substantiate its validity.

Consider the numbers: a study by the IQVIA Institute for Human Data Science indicates a staggering proliferation of health apps, with over 350,000 available across various platforms, a testament to their growing influence. Within these digital tools lies the potential for patients to track symptoms, manage chronic conditions, and even connect with healthcare providers. The primary evidence of their impact is the increased adherence to medication regimens and treatment plans, as reported by the Journal of Medical Internet Research. Patients who use health apps demonstrate a marked improvement in following their prescribed routines, an essential component in the management of chronic illnesses such as diabetes and hypertension.

Yet, to delve deeper is to uncover the layers of how these apps function. They are not mere repositories of information but interactive platforms that engage users through reminders, educational content, and progress tracking. They provide a sense of control, enabling users to visualize changes in their health parameters, thereby reinforcing positive behaviors. And for many, the constant companion of a health app becomes a source of motivation, a digital cheerleader in the pursuit of health goals.

But let us not proceed without caution, for there are counterarguments to consider. Skeptics point out that not all health apps are created equal, and the lack of regulatory oversight raises concerns about the accuracy and reliability of the information they provide. The plethora of choices can overwhelm rather than empower, leading to confusion and potential misuse. Furthermore, the digital divide looms large, questioning the accessibility of such apps to those who may benefit the most yet possess the least resources to engage with them.

In response, it is essential to clarify that while these concerns are valid, they do not diminish the overall positive trajectory of health apps. Regulatory bodies are increasingly recognizing the need for oversight, and initiatives like the FDA's Digital Health Innovation Action Plan are steps toward ensuring that health apps meet stringent standards. Moreover, the acknowledgment of the digital divide has spurred efforts to make health apps more accessible, including designing them for lower-end devices and providing them at reduced or no cost to underserved communities.

Additional supporting evidence of the efficacy of health apps comes from their role in mental health. Amidst the isolation of lockdowns, mental health apps have offered solace and support, connecting users to therapy and resources that might have otherwise been unreachable. This is not an insignificant feat, considering the surge in mental health concerns triggered by the pandemic.

In conclusion, the assertion that health apps have significantly altered the landscape of patient engagement and self-management finds itself reinforced, standing firm against scrutiny. The convergence of technology and healthcare through these apps has provided individuals with unprecedented control over their health journeys, a trend that seems set to continue its upward trajectory. As we navigate the aftermath of a global health crisis, the rise of health apps is a beacon of progress, a reminder that even in the face of adversity, innovation can pave the way for a more empowered and informed society.

Blockchain for Health Data Security

In the evolving narrative of healthcare's metamorphosis, an undercurrent of technological innovation pulses with promise and potential. The sentinel of this transformation is blockchain—a term resonating with intrigue and complexity. As the digital age ushers in an era of unprecedented data exchange, blockchain emerges as a stalwart guardian of information security and privacy, particularly within the sacred realm of health records.

Blockchain technology, often associated with cryptocurrencies like Bitcoin, has steadily gained attention in various industries for its robust security features.

At its core, blockchain is a distributed ledger technology that allows data to be stored in a chain of blocks, each linked and secured using cryptography. This structure ensures that once a piece of information is recorded, it becomes immutable and tamper evident.

A defining characteristic of blockchain is its decentralized nature, which means that no single entity has control over the entire network. This aspect is crucial when considering the sensitivity of health data. Blockchain's inherent design supports transparency and traceability, allowing for a verifiable and auditable trail of all transactions.

The concept of blockchain was first outlined in 1991, but it wasn't until 2008, with the introduction of Bitcoin by an individual or group under the pseudonym Satoshi Nakamoto, that blockchain found its first significant application.

In the healthcare sector, blockchain can be harnessed to create a new standard for data sharing and privacy. It can potentially tackle some of the most persistent challenges in health data management, including interoperability, security, and consent management.

Imagine a healthcare system where patient records are no longer siloed within disparate databases of different healthcare providers. Instead, they are part of a secure, interoperable network where information can be shared quickly, accurately, and with the patient's consent. Blockchain could enable this scenario by providing a platform where each patient's data is encrypted and stored in a way that preserves privacy while still being accessible to authorized parties.

A prevalent misconception is that blockchain is inherently private and anonymous. While blockchain can enhance privacy, it is not anonymous by default; rather, it is pseudonymous, with transactions recorded in a way that they are linked to a specific digital identity.

As the sun sets on the days of simple, unsecured digital records and dawns upon an age where data breaches are a formidable enemy, blockchain stands as a beacon of hope. With the health sector still reeling from the aftershocks of the Covid-19 pandemic, the question arises: How can blockchain technology fortify the walls that safeguard our health data?

Ponder for a moment the magnitude of the challenge. Health records are a trove of sensitive information, a veritable gold mine for malevolent actors seeking to exploit personal data for nefarious purposes. The breach of such data can have dire consequences, ranging from identity theft to insurance fraud. Hence, the imperative to secure health data is not merely a technical concern—it is a moral one.

Diving deeper into the mechanics of blockchain, we find that each block in the chain contains a hash—a unique digital fingerprint—of the preceding block, alongside its own hash and timestamp. If an attempt to alter a record is made, the hash would change, and the network would quickly spot this anomaly. The alteration of one block would necessitate the alteration of all subsequent blocks, a task so computationally intensive that it is considered virtually impossible.

Yet, the canvas of blockchain is not monochromatic. There are different types of blockchains: public, private, and consortium, each with varying degrees of openness and permission. In healthcare, private or consortium blockchains are more appropriate, as they restrict who can participate in the network, thus offering an additional layer of privacy and security.

Striding through the gallery of blockchain applications, we encounter smart contracts—self-executing contracts with the terms of the agreement directly written into code. In healthcare, smart contracts could automate consent management, ensuring that patients' data is shared only when they have granted explicit permission, thus upholding the principle of patient autonomy.

However, as with any technology, blockchain is not a panacea. It introduces new complexities. For instance, the question of how to correct erroneous information without undermining the integrity of the ledger remains a subject of debate. The immutability of blockchain is a double-edged sword, providing security but complicating corrections.

In the realm of vivid imagery, envisage a healthcare system that operates with the fluidity and precision of a symphony, each player—the patients, providers, payers—orchestrated by the maestro of blockchain technology. Data flows seamlessly, and privacy is not a concern whispered in hushed tones but a robust reality.

As we march toward this future, blockchain in healthcare remains a burgeoning field, ripe with potential yet grounded in the sobriety of its challenges. It is not a question of if blockchain will alter the landscape of health data security, but rather, how and when. The curtain has been drawn back, revealing the silhouette of a future where health data security is not an oxymoron but a tangible, achievable aspiration.

For those who stand at the crossroads of technology and healthcare, ponder this: Can we afford to ignore the clarion call of blockchain, or will we embrace its potential and redefine the sanctity of our health records? The path forward is not just a technical journey but a collective leap of faith into a domain where the guardianship of our most personal data is not just an expectation, but a reality etched into the very blocks of our digital existence.

Chapter Four

Patient Experience and Engagement

Virtual Waiting Rooms

In the heart of a bustling city, there once was a clinic that stood as a testament to the relentless pursuit of medical excellence. As one navigates through its corridors, which have been witness to countless stories of human resilience, a transformation subtle yet profound quietly unfolded in the wake of the global pandemic.

Dr. Eleanor Voss, a seasoned physician, and her team at the Harmony Health Clinic were at the forefront of this metamorphosis. Harmony Health, known for its patient-centric approach, faced an unprecedented challenge as the world grappled with the Covid-19 crisis. The waiting room, once a hive of activity with the hum of conversation and the rustle of magazine pages, stood eerily silent and empty.

The core challenge was clear: How could the clinic maintain its commitment to patient care while adhering to the strict social distancing mandates? The answer lay in an innovative leap into the digital realm – the virtual waiting room.

The approach was multifaceted. Harmony Health invested in robust telehealth platforms, trained staff to navigate the new digital landscape, and developed protocols to manage patient flow virtually. They partnered with tech companies to create a seamless check-in process that patients could complete from the safety of their homes or cars.

As patients logged in, they were greeted by virtual receptionists – friendly faces on screens offering the same warmth as in-person interactions. Physicians like Dr. Voss would then consult with patients via video calls, ensuring that the standard of care remained uncompromised.

The results were telling. Patient satisfaction scores soared – no longer were they bound by the constraints of travel or the anxiety of crowded spaces. Data showed a marked decrease in no-show rates and an increase in the timeliness of appointments.

But it wasn't just about the data. It was about the stories – like that of an elderly gentleman who could now discuss his health concerns without the physical toll of a clinic visit or the young mother who could receive postnatal advice while her newborn slept peacefully beside her.

Reflecting on this journey, there were valuable lessons to be learned. The digital divide became evident as some patients struggled to navigate the new technology. The team had to innovate constantly to ensure inclusivity, offering phone consultations and setting up community kiosks for those without internet access.

Visual aids, such as step-by-step guides and videos demonstrating the use of the telehealth platform, were developed to enhance patient understanding and comfort with the technology.

This shift to virtual waiting rooms was more than a mere response to a crisis; it was an evolution in the very essence of healthcare delivery. It is connected to the larger narrative of a world where digital and physical realities merge to create more accessible and personalized healthcare experiences.

And so, one might ponder, what does the future hold for the traditional waiting room? Will the soothing pastel walls and rows of chairs become relics of a bygone era?

As I, Alexander Ruche, reflect on my time in the IMCU during the pandemic, I can attest to the resilience and adaptability of healthcare workers. The virtual waiting room is just one example of the countless innovations that have reshaped the landscape of healthcare.

Perhaps, then, the question is not whether healthcare has changed, but how we, as providers and patients alike, continue to evolve with it. How do we harness the power of technology to enhance, not replace, the human touch that is the cornerstone of healing?

Let us step into the next chapter with the wisdom of our experiences, the courage to innovate, and the unwavering commitment to care that defines us.

The virtual waiting room, while a symbol of change, is ultimately a reminder of our capacity to reimagine and reinvent in the face of adversity. It is a testament to the enduring spirit of healthcare – a spirit that cannot, even in the darkest of times, be extinguished.

Patient Education and Covid-19

In the shadow of the pandemic, a new chapter in healthcare emerged like a phoenix rising from the ashes of uncertainty. It was not just about adapting to change; it was about revolutionizing the very fabric of patient interaction and education. The virus, invisible yet insidious, demanded a response that was not only swift but also enduring. It called for a bridge to be built between knowledge and behavior, a conduit through which patient education could flow and alter the landscape of public health.

Understanding the gravity of the situation, the healthcare community embarked on a mission to empower patients with knowledge, transforming them from passive recipients of care to informed partners in the battle against Covid-19. This was not just an adaptation; it was a revolution in patient education, marking a turn in the tides of healthcare.

The goal was to create an informed patient populace, armed with the knowledge to not only protect themselves but also to prevent the spread of the virus. But how would this be achieved?

The prerequisites were clear: accurate information, accessible platforms for dissemination, and a populace willing to learn. The healthcare professionals needed to be educators, the internet a classroom, and every piece of communication a lesson in preventive health behavior.

A broad overview of this initiative included developing educational materials, utilizing multiple communication channels, and continuously updating information as our understanding of the virus evolved.

Focusing in, the first step was creating clear, concise, and accurate educational content. This content ranged from the symptoms of Covid-19 to the importance of handwashing, social distancing, and mask-wearing. It also included information on what to do if one suspects they have the virus, how to get tested, and the nuances of contact tracing.

Practical advice was woven into these materials. Tips on proper mask-wearing, effective handwashing techniques, and protocols for self-isolation were shared. Warnings about the dangers of misinformation and the importance of relying on credible sources were emphasized.

To validate the success of these efforts, metrics such as the reduction in infection rates, the number of individuals engaging with the educational materials, and feedback from the community were monitored closely.

Yet, challenges persisted. Misinformation led to confusion and fear. To troubleshoot this, healthcare providers doubled down on their efforts to communicate clearly and correct fallacies with evidence-based information.

The silhouette of the pandemic loomed large, yet it was met with a resilience that was both inspiring and instructive. As healthcare providers, the question begged to be asked: how do we maintain this momentum of patient education beyond the crisis? How do we ensure that the lessons learned are not confined to the history books but are carried forward to forge a healthcare system that is more robust and patient-informed?

The answer lies in the integration of these educational strategies into the very DNA of healthcare. It requires a commitment to not only treat but also educate, to see the patient as a whole – a person with the capacity to understand and participate in their own health journey.

Let me paint you a picture: Imagine a world where every patient feels equipped to make informed decisions about their health, where doctors are not just healers but also teachers, and where the healthcare system is not a labyrinth but a clear path to wellness.

This is not a fanciful dream. It is the legacy of Covid-19 – a virus that changed the world and, in doing so, changed healthcare forever.

In conclusion, the evolution of patient education during the Covid-19 pandemic is not just a footnote in the annals of healthcare history. It is a beacon that guides us toward a future where empowered patients stand side by side with healthcare providers to create a healthier, more informed world. It is a testament to human tenacity and the unwavering spirit of innovation that has always been at the heart of medicine.

The journey of patient education in the era of Covid-19 is a mosaic of courage, innovation, and foresight. It is a narrative that weaves together the threads of knowledge, technology, and human compassion. As we turn the page on this chapter, let us carry with us the lessons it has taught us, for they are the map to a brighter, healthier tomorrow.

The Shift to Outpatient Care

In the wake of a global health emergency, the landscape of medical care underwent a seismic shift. The Covid-19 pandemic, a crisis of unfathomable scale, acted as a catalyst for change, thrusting the healthcare system into a new era where outpatient services and home recovery became the vanguard of patient care. This shift to outpatient care was not born out of the pandemic, but its roots can be traced back to a burgeoning trend that the crisis simply expedited.

Outpatient care, a term once synonymous with minor treatments and quick consultations, evolved into a complex system capable of supporting a wide range of medical services, from diagnostics to post-operative care. But what sparked this evolution, and how did it gain such momentum during the pandemic?

Consider the earliest origins of outpatient services. They began as an ancillary function of hospitals, offering a venue for treatments that did not require an overnight stay. This system saw incremental improvements over the years, with technological advancements and a growing emphasis on patient convenience driving the expansion of services offered in these settings.

As we chronicle the major milestones, we observe the integration of telemedicine, the rise of ambulatory surgery centers, and the increasing sophistication of home health care services. Each of these developments played a pivotal role in establishing the robust outpatient care infrastructure we know today.

The onset of the pandemic thrust this infrastructure into the spotlight. With hospitals becoming battlegrounds against the virus, the need to manage patient flow and minimize exposure risk became critical. Outpatient services offered a solution, allowing for continuity of care while alleviating the strain on inpatient facilities.

Visualize, if you will, the bustling corridors of a hospital, now quieted, its usual patients now receiving care in the comfort of their own homes. Technology bridged the gap, with virtual consultations and remote monitoring becoming commonplace. This image reflects a profound transformation, an adaptation born out of necessity that has since become a mainstay in the healthcare paradigm.

Such transformations, however, were not uniform across the globe. Cultural and regional variations dictated the pace and nature of this shift. In some areas, pre-existing telehealth platforms allowed for a seamless transition, while in others, the lack of infrastructure posed significant challenges. Yet, the direction was clear—outpatient care was to play a decisive role in the future of healthcare delivery.

As we delve into modern interpretations and adaptations, we uncover a landscape teeming with innovation. From mobile health clinics to sophisticated home care kits, the tools and services available to patients are more advanced and accessible than ever before. The Covid-19 pandemic has not only accelerated these trends but has also ingrained them into the very fabric of healthcare.

But the journey has not been without its obstacles. Controversies around quality of care, data privacy, and the digital divide have sparked debate. The turning point came with the realization that these challenges must be addressed head-on, through policy reform, education, and investment in technology.

Now, let us pose a direct question: In this era of rapid change, how do we ensure that the quality of outpatient care matches, or even surpasses, that of traditional inpatient services? The answer lies in ongoing innovation, stringent quality controls, and a patient-centered approach that prioritizes accessibility and outcomes.

In this new dawn of healthcare, we witness the emergence of patients as active participants in their care. They are no longer mere visitors to a doctor's office but are now empowered individuals managing their health from the comfort of their homes. This fundamental change in perspective is a testament to the lasting impact of the pandemic on healthcare.

To truly convey the essence of this evolution, let us share a story. Picture an elderly man, once bound by the need for frequent hospital visits, now engaging with his physician through a tablet, receiving care that is both personal and precise. This is not just a convenience; it is a revolution that redefines patient autonomy and dignity.

The shift to outpatient care, as we have seen, is not a temporary response to an unprecedented crisis. It is a permanent reimagining of how healthcare is delivered, experienced, and perceived. It stands as a powerful reminder that in the face of adversity, innovation can forge paths to a future that once seemed out of reach.

In sum, the story of outpatient care during and beyond the Covid-19 pandemic is one of agility, resilience, and foresight. It is a narrative that continues to unfold, driven by the collective will to create a healthcare system that is not only responsive to the needs of the moment but also anticipatory of the challenges of tomorrow. This is the legacy of a pandemic that reshaped our world and the healthcare system that rose to meet it—a system forever changed, forever forward-moving.

Health Literacy in a Pandemic

As dawn light filters through the blinds of a quiet suburban home, a middle-aged woman sits at her kitchen table, a steaming cup of coffee in hand, and a smartphone displaying a health app by her side. It's a serene picture, and yet, it belies an underlying tension—a reflection of the informational maelstrom that has gripped our world since the emergence of Covid-19. In this new reality, where medical advice is sought with the swipe of a finger, the urgency for clear and accurate health communication has never been more critical.

Delving into the heart of the matter, we must confront a stark reality: the pandemic has laid bare the complexities of conveying crucial health information to a diverse public. From mask-wearing guidelines to vaccination protocols, the task of disseminating data that is both digestible and scientifically sound has proven daunting.

What happens when such vital messaging falls short of its mark? The consequences are grave—misinformation can spread like wildfire, eroding public trust and compromising safety measures. Without intervention, the very fabric of public health could unravel, leaving communities vulnerable and healthcare systems overwhelmed.

In the quest for a solution, we turn to the cornerstone of crisis communication: health literacy. Imagine, if you will, a world where every individual—regardless of education or background—grasps the implications of public health directives and can make informed decisions for themselves and their loved ones. It's a lofty goal, but not unattainable.

The implementation of this vision begins with simplification. Medical jargon, that oft-impenetrable lexicon, must be translated into everyday language. Infographics, visual aids, and even storytelling can serve as powerful tools to illuminate complex concepts.

But how do we ensure that these strategies truly penetrate the psyche of a diverse populace? The process involves a multilayered approach: health authorities collaborating with community leaders, educators, and even local influencers to tailor messages that resonate across cultural and socioeconomic divides.

Consider the story of a small town that rallied together to combat vaccine hesitancy. Enlisting the help of the local barber, a trusted figure with the gift of gab, they transformed his shop into a hub of conversation and education. The barber, armed with facts and a comforting presence, became an ambassador for health literacy, his shop a microcosm of the community-centric approach needed on a grander scale.

Drawing from such grassroots initiatives, we anticipate a ripple effect, where success stories bolster the broader effort to enhance health literacy. But where is the evidence to support this optimism? Research attests to the efficacy of community engagement in public health campaigns, with increased comprehension and compliance observed among populations exposed to targeted messaging.

Yet, in the spirit of comprehensive discourse, we must acknowledge that alternative solutions exist. Digital platforms offer interactive learning experiences, while traditional media campaigns cast wide nets of influence. Each method possesses unique merits and limitations, prompting a blend of strategies to achieve optimal outcomes.

Are you, dear reader, prepared to navigate this intricate web of health communication? It's a challenge that demands unwavering dedication, creativity, and empathy. By embracing simplicity in language, harnessing the power of visuals, and fostering community connections, we can bridge the gap between medical knowledge and public understanding—a bridge that not only withstands the torrents of a pandemic but also carries us towards a future of empowered, health-literate societies.

In conclusion, the transformation of healthcare in the wake of Covid-19 is not confined to the physical realm of hospitals and clinics. It extends to the sphere of information, where the battle for clarity and comprehension is fought daily. As we continue to chart this uncharted territory, let us hold fast to the belief that through collaboration, innovation, and unwavering commitment to public education, we can change the landscape of health literacy, and in doing so, safeguard the wellbeing of generations to come.

Patient Autonomy and Informed Consent

Embark on a journey that promises to revolutionize your understanding of healthcare in the post-pandemic world. As you turn the pages of this book, you will discover the delicate balance between urgency and patient rights—a balance that has never been more critical than in the wake of Covid-19. I, Alexander Ruche, a nurse on the frontlines, will guide you through the intricate dance of swift action and informed consent, revealing how the pandemic has reshaped our approach to patient autonomy.

The methodologies laid out in this narrative are not just theoretical musings. They are the byproducts of countless hours spent in the IMCU, where split-second decisions often clashed with the need for thorough patient understanding. You will gain insights into the emergency protocols that had to be reimagined, the communication strategies that were overhauled, and the ethical challenges we bravely faced.

You might wonder, how can we ensure patient rights when the world is spinning in a health crisis? How do we balance informed consent with the necessity of immediate action? These are valid doubts, and they will not be dismissed. Instead, they will be meticulously dismantled, piece by piece, as we explore the evolution of patient care protocols during the pandemic.

Picture a healthcare landscape where every patient is not only a passive recipient of care but an active participant in their treatment journey. This vision, once a distant dream, has been drawn closer to reality by the forceful tide of Covid-19. Your eyes will be opened to the transformative power of clear communication, the newfound respect for patient autonomy, and the robust systems established to ensure that every voice is heard even amidst chaos.

As you delve deeper into this book, your commitment to understanding the new healthcare paradigm will be solidified. The value of what lies ahead is not just in the acquisition of knowledge but in the life-changing potential it holds for healthcare providers and patients alike. The lessons from the pandemic are not fleeting; they are the bedrock of a forever altered healthcare terrain.

The seeds of change were sown in the heart of the crisis. In the IMCU, we were faced with the daunting task of treating patients who were not just fighting for their lives but also grappling with the fear and uncertainty that came with a novel virus. It was here that the essence of patient autonomy and informed consent was tested, and ultimately, strengthened.

Imagine, for a moment, the tumultuous early days of the pandemic. Visitation restrictions meant patients were often alone, making decisions without the immediate support of loved ones. We had to find new ways to ensure that they were fully informed and comfortable with the care they were receiving. Virtual conferencing, simplified consent forms, and more accessible information were just the beginning. These innovations were not mere stopgaps; they evolved into permanent fixtures, enhancing patient engagement and empowerment.

Yet, the path to this enhanced engagement was not straightforward. We wrestled with questions that had no easy answers. How do you convey the risks of an experimental treatment to a critically ill patient? How much information is enough, and how much is overwhelming? These questions forced us to reevaluate our approach, to ensure that even in the most pressing situations, the patient's voice remained paramount.

In this book, you will find stories of real people, like the young man who, despite the severity of his condition, was given the chance to understand and consent to an experimental therapy. His courage and the trust he placed in us to respect his autonomy became a beacon, illuminating the importance of our mission.

Some might say that the crisis demanded shortcuts around patient autonomy. I argue the opposite. It demanded more from us—more attention to detail, more compassion, more dedication to the principles of informed consent.

And so, we adapted. We learned to convey complex information quickly and compassionately. We embraced technologies that bridged gaps between patient and provider. We honed our ability to listen, truly listen, to the fears and desires of those in our care.

This book does not avoid the uncomfortable truths. It acknowledges the missteps and the learning curves. But it also celebrates the victories, small and large, in our pursuit of a healthcare system that respects the rights and wisdom of patients.

You may ask, "What now? What does the future hold for patient autonomy?" The answer lies in the chapters to come, where we explore the lasting impact of our pandemic experiences on the relationship between healthcare providers and patients.

In closing, let us not forget the resilience and adaptability that have been hallmarks of this unprecedented time. The ways in which Covid changed healthcare are myriad, but the enhancement of patient autonomy and informed consent stands as a testament to the strength of the human spirit in the face of adversity. Join me as we continue to explore how these changes have shaped a new era of healthcare—one that honors the agency and dignity of every individual.

Chapter Five

Global Health Dynamics

Pandemic's Impact on Global Health Equity

In the early months of 2020, a virus invisible to the naked eye laid bare the vast chasms that exist within global health equity. One staggering revelation emerged: the wealthiest 10% of nations accounted for more than 75% of all COVID-19 vaccinations administered by mid-2021, while the poorest countries languished with barely 2% of their populations receiving a single dose. This is not just a number; it is a testament to a world divided, a world where the accident of birthplace dictates one's chance at health, at survival.

Why should this matter to us? Because in the intricate web of global interconnectedness, the health of the individual in the farthest corner of the earth impacts the well-being of every one of us. When a virus can travel from one side of the globe to the other in less than a day, no one is safe until everyone is safe. The stark inequality in health care access is not just a moral failure; it's a direct threat to global health security.

As a nurse who served in an Intermediate Care Unit (IMCU) throughout the entire pandemic, I witnessed firsthand the harrowing disparities that COVID-19 both exposed and exacerbated. The narrative that unfolds in the chapters of this book is not just an academic discourse; it's a mosaic of real-life stories, a tapestry woven from the threads of human experience during the most defining health crisis of our generation.

What can we learn from this? What unseen depths of systemic failure does this pandemic reveal? How can we emerge not only with a resolve to heal but with tangible strategies to ensure equitable health care for all? This book seeks to answer these questions, delving into the heart of what it means to be part of a global community in the face of a crisis.

How, you might ask, did such disparities come to be? The narrative often paints a picture of resource scarcity, but is that the complete truth? Could it be that our global health system is built on a foundation of inequality, one that favors the wealthy and neglects the poor? This book dares to peel back the layers of this complex issue, revealing a confluence of factors that range from patent laws and pharmaceutical monopolies to the logistical challenges of delivering healthcare in remote regions.

In this revelatory journey, we'll explore the stories of those who fought on the front lines, the patients who faced the brunt of this inequity, and the policymakers who grappled with decisions that would impact millions. Each account provides a unique vantage point, a piece of the puzzle that, when assembled, presents a clear picture of the monumental task at hand.

What if the solution lies not only in the hands of governments and international bodies but also within the realm of local communities and individual action? Could a grassroots approach to healthcare equity, one that empowers local leaders and leverages innovation, be the key to a more just world?

The world stood still as the pandemic swept through nations, leaving a trail of death, despair, and a profound sense of urgency to rectify the wrongs of our healthcare systems. It is a wake-up call that cannot be unheeded.

"Healthcare for all" – this phrase took on a new, desperate meaning as emergency rooms overflowed, ventilators ran in short supply, and vaccines became the new currency of survival. It's a call to action that reverberates through the pages of this book, a clarion call to redefine what we accept as the norm in global health.

As we bridge from the initial shock of these revelations to the enlightening journey ahead, let us ask ourselves: How can we foster a world where every human being, regardless of geography or economic status, has a fair chance at health and wellbeing? How do we dismantle the barriers that obstruct this vision of equity?

This book does not claim to have all the answers, but it endeavors to shine a light on the path forward. Through the lens of my experiences as a nurse, the insights of experts, and the voices of the marginalized, we will navigate the complexities of a world forever changed by a pandemic. A world where the lessons learned must pave the way for a more equitable future.

The path ahead is fraught with challenges, but it is also ripe with opportunity. The solutions we seek may not be easy, nor will they be quick, but they are necessary. Together, let us embark on this crucial journey – a journey toward healing, toward unity, and toward a world where health equity is not an ideal, but a reality.

International Supply Chain for PPE

Amidst the chaos of a world grappling with an unprecedented health crisis, the unassuming heroes emerged not just in hospitals and clinics but also on factory floors, in warehouses, and at border crossings. The demand for personal protective equipment (PPE) skyrocketed as the COVID-19 pandemic unfurled across continents, painting a stark image of urgency and scarcity that would forever alter the landscape of healthcare and its intricate supply chains.

As dawn broke over the sprawling industrial hubs of Asia, the hum of machinery blended with the anxious voices of logistics coordinators. Countries worldwide were waking up to a reality where the protection of frontline workers hinged on the seamless operation of these facilities. But the scene was far from tranquil. Orders piled up, factories stretched to their limits, and the fragility of a system that underpins global health security was laid bare.

The players in this unfolding drama were as diverse as the nations they served. Manufacturers, freight carriers, government bodies, and healthcare institutions, all thrust into a frenetic dance of supply and demand. The challenge was monumental: to equip every nurse, doctor, and healthcare worker with adequate PPE to combat an invisible adversary that was claiming lives at an alarming rate.

Beneath the surface of this logistical endeavor was a convoluted web of policies, trade agreements, and economic interests. Countries faced export bans, import restrictions, and bidding wars that turned allies into competitors. In the eye of this storm, the mission was clear – ensure that PPE reached those who needed it most, without delay.

The strategies employed were as varied as they were ingenious. Manufacturers pivoted production lines overnight, fashioning respirators out of snorkeling masks and gowns out of industrial materials. Governments and private entities formed alliances, sharing information and resources to streamline distribution. Innovators harnessed the power of technology, creating open-source designs for 3D printed face shields and ventilator parts.

The results, while mixed, bore testimony to human resilience and adaptability. Some regions saw an influx of PPE, stabilizing their healthcare systems amidst surging cases. Others struggled, hampered by logistical nightmares and ineffective coordination. The stories of success were heartening; those of failure, a grim reminder of the work that lay ahead.

Reflecting on these tumultuous times, one cannot ignore the lessons etched into the very fabric of global healthcare. The need for robust, transparent, and responsive supply chains has never been more evident. The reliance on a few countries for critical supplies came under scrutiny, pushing for a renaissance in local manufacturing capabilities.

Yet, amidst the charts and graphs that attempt to capture the essence of this crisis, the human element remains paramount. The image of a solitary healthcare worker donning a fresh mask, a barrier of hope against an unseen foe, is a powerful one. It speaks to the collective effort that spanned continents and industries, a testament to the spirit of cooperation that COVID-19 unwittingly ignited.

How, then, does this narrative fold back into the larger tapestry of a healthcare system transformed by a pandemic? The answer lies in the recognition of our interconnectedness and the acknowledgment that no nation, no individual, stands in isolation. The supply chain for PPE is but one thread in the vast and intricate weave of global health.

As we turn the page on this case study and gaze toward the horizon, a question lingers – what other challenges await us in a post-pandemic world? How will we harness the lessons learned to fortify our defenses against the next global threat?

In these reflections, we find not the end, but the beginning of a dialogue. A conversation that extends beyond the confines of this book and into the halls of power, the communities we serve, and the very heart of our shared human experience.

For as long as pathogens exist, the need for protection will persist. The international supply chain for PPE, once an overlooked cog in the machinery of healthcare, has emerged as a critical lifeline – one that must be nurtured, strengthened, and respected. Our collective health, as the COVID-19 pandemic has irrevocably proven, depends on it.

Lessons From Different Healthcare Models

In the tapestry of healthcare, the pandemic's thread has been woven in dark hues, a reminder of the vulnerability of even the most robust systems. It has brought into sharp relief the stark contrasts and surprising parallels between different healthcare models across the globe. In this chapter, we delve into the heart of these systems, analyzing how various nations responded to the COVID-19 crisis and what it means for the future of healthcare.

The pandemic served as an unplanned experiment, one that tested the resilience, adaptability, and efficiency of healthcare infrastructures. At the heart of this analysis lies a crucial question: What can we learn from these disparate approaches to healthcare, and how might these lessons alter the course of medical practice forever?

To commence this exploration, we must consider the criteria for our comparison. The benchmarks include, but are not limited to, the accessibility of healthcare services, the speed and effectiveness of the response, the capacity for innovation, and the overall outcomes in terms of infection rates and mortality.

When we juxtapose two seemingly dissimilar healthcare models — the centralized, state-funded systems typical of many European countries with the mixed-market models like that of the United States — we uncover a mosaic of responses that challenge preconceived notions. Did universal healthcare offer the silver bullet, or did the agility of private-sector-driven models prove superior?

The similarities, at first glance, may seem scarce, yet they exist. Across the board, healthcare providers showed an unprecedented level of commitment and bravery. Systems, regardless of their underlying principles, had to pivot and adapt, embracing telemedicine and digital health platforms. The shared goal was clear: to mitigate the spread of the virus and provide care to the afflicted.

Contrasts, however, were more pronounced. Countries with centralized healthcare models could marshal resources and coordinate responses more uniformly, leveraging the power of a single governing body. In contrast, mixed-market systems faced challenges in unifying the approach, with disparities in access and outcomes more evident.

Visual aids, such as graphs and charts, are not mere embellishments; they serve as stark illustrations of these comparisons. They depict the trajectories of infection curves, the capacity of hospital beds, and the speed of vaccine rollouts, offering a clear-eyed view of each system's efficacy.

But what do these comparisons reveal? A complex tapestry of cause and effect. Centralized systems, while sometimes sluggish to innovate, provided a safety net for the most vulnerable. Mixed-market models, on the other hand, demonstrated bursts of innovation and resourcefulness, though often at the cost of uniformity and equity.

The broader implications are profound. The pandemic has exposed the need for flexibility in healthcare, for systems that can quickly pivot and adapt to crisis. It has highlighted the importance of universal health coverage, as populations with easier access to care often fared better. It has also underscored the critical role of public health and the need for investment in preventative measures.

Moving beyond theory, these lessons have real-world relevance. As we emerge from the shadow of COVID-19, governments are re-evaluating their healthcare policies. There is a palpable shift towards systems that blend the best of both worlds: the efficiency and innovation of the private sector with the coverage and equity of public health services.

What does this mean for you, the reader? Have you noticed a change in the way healthcare is delivered in your community? Have you experienced firsthand the benefits of telehealth or the frustration of a strained public health system?

In this narrative, every one of us plays a role. The decisions we advocate for, the policies we support, and the way we value healthcare workers will shape the post-pandemic world. The lessons learned are not merely academic; they are the blueprint for a future where healthcare is more accessible, more resilient, and more attuned to the needs of every individual.

In conclusion, the pandemic has been both a mirror and a catalyst, reflecting the flaws and strengths of different healthcare models while propelling us towards systemic change. It is up to us to carry forward the insights gleaned from this tumultuous period, ensuring that the healthcare systems of tomorrow are not only prepared for the next global health challenge but are also more equitable, just, and humane. This is our collective responsibility, and it is one we must embrace with both urgency and hope.

The Role of WHO and CDC

In the dense fog of uncertainty that enveloped the world as a novel coronavirus emerged, two organizations stood as beacons of guidance and authority: the World Health Organization (WHO) and the Centers for Disease Control and Prevention (CDC). Their directives and insights would come to shape the turbulent months and years that followed, steering the course of the pandemic's narrative.

Let us cast our minds back to a time before this global health crisis, to the inception of these pivotal institutions. The WHO, born from the ashes of war in 1948, was mandated to direct and coordinate international health within the United Nations' system. The CDC's roots stretch even further back to 1946, initially focusing on malaria control in war-torn areas of the United States before expanding its reach to a plethora of public health challenges. These historical milestones, set decades apart, were the progenitors of a new era in global and national health governance.

Fast forward to the present, and the roles of the WHO and CDC have expanded exponentially. They have become the architects of disease prevention and response strategies, with their expertise sought after in every corner of the globe. But why look to the past when the present crisis demands our attention? Because history is the greatest teacher, and its lessons are invaluable in navigating the present and sculpting a better future.

The COVID-19 pandemic was not the first test for these organizations, nor will it be the last. Yet, it was unprecedented in its scale and the modern interconnectedness it exploited, presenting challenges that no single nation could tackle alone. The WHO and CDC found themselves at the forefront of a war against an invisible enemy, one that required a coordinated, comprehensive international response.

In those early days, the WHO emerged as a global harbinger of information, disseminating data about the virus's spread and providing guidelines for containment and mitigation. The CDC, concurrently, played a critical role within the United States, offering expertise and recommendations to shape the national response. Both organizations faced immense pressure and scrutiny as the pandemic unfolded, with their every decision impacting millions.

Have you ever wondered how these organizations managed to stay abreast of the rapidly evolving situation? They harnessed decades of experience and the collective knowledge of countless professionals who worked tirelessly behind the scenes. Their collaborative efforts were a testament to the power of unity in the face of adversity.

As the virus spread with alacrity, both the WHO and CDC had to swiftly adapt their strategies. It was a colossal undertaking: tracking the virus, advising on public health measures, coordinating with governments, and eventually, guiding the development and distribution of life-saving vaccines. Their historic role in this pandemic will be analyzed and debated for years to come.

Why does this matter now? In a post-pandemic world, the actions and decisions of these organizations continue to resonate. They have set precedents, crafted new paradigms for disease control, and underscored the necessity of preparedness and cooperation. Their influence extends beyond the confines of health departments and into the very fabric of society.

As we transition from the historical context to the contemporary expanse of healthcare, it's clear that the WHO and CDC have not only directed the battle against COVID-19 but have also catalyzed a transformation in healthcare. Their guidance during the pandemic has redefined public health policies, shaped the development of telemedicine, and pushed the boundaries of vaccine research and distribution.

With each chapter of this unfolding story, we witness the evolution of healthcare under the aegis of these organizations. And so, we find ourselves at a pivotal moment, at the nexus of past experience and future innovation. The story of how the WHO and CDC have shaped the healthcare landscape is far from over; it continues to be written with each new development, each policy adjustment, and each life touched by their influence.

As the reader embarks on this journey through the chapters of change, one should ponder the gravity of the WHO and CDC's roles. How have their actions impacted your understanding of health and disease? How will their guidance influence the way we prepare for and respond to future health crises?

The pandemic may have altered the course of history, but it has also amplified the significance of robust health organizations. The lessons learned from COVID-19, and the role of the WHO and CDC, will indelibly mark the pages of healthcare for generations to come. As we forge ahead, let us carry with us the knowledge that in unity and informed action lies the strength to overcome even the most formidable health challenges.

Vaccine Diplomacy and Geopolitics

With a career deeply rooted in the heart of healthcare, my voice carries with it the weight of firsthand experience and a profound understanding of the complexities that underpin our global health systems. My name is Alexander Ruche, and I have dedicated my life to nursing—a profession that not only demands technical proficiency but also an unwavering commitment to human welfare. As an integral part of an Intermediate Care Unit (IMCU) team throughout the entirety of the

COVID-19 pandemic, I witnessed the unfolding of a crisis that would forever alter the landscape of healthcare and international relations.

My journey began long before this pandemic, in the bustling hallways of hospitals where every decision could tip the scales between life and death. The years I spent honing my skills at the bedside of the critically ill equipped me with a deep-seated knowledge of patient care and the inner workings of health institutions. It was during these formative years that I cultivated a perspective on healthcare that transcends borders, recognizing early on that the health of one is inexorably linked to the health of all.

The laurels I bear are not merely symbols of individual achievement but reflect a lifelong pursuit of excellence and innovation in nursing. They serve as a testament to my role as an educator, a leader in healthcare policy discussions, and an advocate for equitable access to medical resources. My accolades, while humbling, have never been the end goal; they are milestones on a path that I tread with the conviction that knowledge must be shared and used as a catalyst for change.

Perhaps the most poignant chapter in my narrative is the personal investment I made during the height of the pandemic. The scenes of desperation, the faces of my colleagues etched with fatigue, and the collective yearning for a reprieve from the relentless tide of illness—these are imprinted upon my soul. It was a time that demanded resilience, an unwavering spirit, and above all, a sense of duty that extended beyond the hospital walls. It is from this crucible of challenge that I draw my resolve to contribute to a broader discourse—one that encompasses the geopolitical ramifications of a health crisis.

As we turn the page to the present discussion, I invite you to partake in an exploration of a facet of the pandemic that is as consequential as it is contentious—vaccine diplomacy and geopolitics. This book is not just a recounting of events; it is an invitation to understand the political dimensions of vaccine distribution and the intricate dance of international relations that it has entailed.

Why is this conversation important now, you may ask? Because the reverberations of vaccine diplomacy are still being felt across the globe, shaping alliances and creating fissures that will influence geopolitical landscapes for years to come. Have you considered how the availability of a vaccine in one country over another speaks volumes about power, influence, and the priorities of nations?

The distribution of COVID-19 vaccines has become a theater where geopolitical interests play out, where the aspirations of nations to assert their dominance or to foster alliances come into sharp relief. Nations with vaccine manufacturing capabilities have found themselves in positions of power, able to leverage their resources for strategic gains. But what of the nation's left waiting, their populations vulnerable and their pleas for equity echoing in the halls of power?

I have seen the faces of those who waited, their hopes pinned on the promise of protection that a vaccine represents. And I have grappled with the ethical implications of a world where life-saving medical interventions become pawns in a larger game of influence and control.

In this chapter, I delve into the intricate dance of vaccine diplomacy, unveiling the strategic moves and countermoves that have characterized this new frontier. We will explore the alliances forged in the pursuit of vaccine equity, the quiet tensions that simmer beneath the surface, and the profound questions that arise when health becomes intertwined with national interests.

As you journey through this narrative, I challenge you to think critically about the implications of vaccine diplomacy on global health security. What does it mean for the future of pandemic preparedness? How do we navigate the delicate balance between national self-interest and collective good? And how can we, as a global community, ensure that the lessons learned from this pandemic pave the way for a more equitable and resilient healthcare system?

This book is more than a chronicle of the past; it is a blueprint for the future. It is a call to action for those who hold the levers of power and for every individual who believes in the sanctity of health as a human right. Together, let us embark on this journey of enlightenment, armed with the knowledge that our collective future hinges on the decisions we make today.

Chapter Six

Mental Health and Resilience

Coping Strategies for Healthcare Workers

In the shadowed corridors of hospitals and clinics, the healthcare workers who once moved with unflagging purpose now navigate an ever-shifting landscape, one irrevocably altered by the global Covid pandemic. These tireless individuals, often hailed as heroes, face an onslaught of new stresses and challenges, pressing the need for effective coping strategies into the forefront of the dialogue surrounding healthcare reform.

Before the dawn of this unprecedented era, the healthcare system was already a crucible of high-pressure situations. Yet, in the wake of Covid, the intensity has magnified, and the stakes have soared. It is within this context that we consider a vital compendium of strategies, designed to safeguard the well-being of these essential warriors in the medical field. The importance of this list cannot be overstated; it serves as a beacon for those adrift in the tumultuous seas of post-pandemic healthcare.

The following represent the cornerstones of resilience and mental fortitude:

1. Mindfulness and Meditation
2. Physical Activity and Exercise
3. Adequate Rest and Sleep Hygiene
4. Professional Counseling and Peer Support
5. Work-life Balance and Time Management
6. Continuous Education and Skill Development

In the heart of chaos, mindfulness emerges as an oasis of tranquility. It is the art of anchoring oneself to the present moment, a skill that, when honed, can act as a bulwark against the tempest of stressors endemic to healthcare settings. Meditation, its close relative, offers a structured path to achieve this centered state of being.

The principles of mindfulness teach practitioners to observe their thoughts and feelings without judgment, thus diminishing the impact of negative emotions. Meditation, often through guided sessions or focused breathing exercises, facilitates a deeper exploration of one's inner landscape, promoting relaxation and clarity of mind.

Studies have consistently shown that healthcare professionals who engage in regular mindfulness practices report lower levels of stress and anxiety. Dr. Emma Richardson, a seasoned ER nurse, shares, "Starting my day with just ten minutes of meditation has made an overwhelming difference. It's like I've been given a shield against the day's unpredictability."

Implementing short, daily mindfulness exercises can significantly mitigate the effects of burnout. Even during a busy shift, taking a moment to breathe deeply and refocus can reset a frayed nervous system.

The benefits of regular physical activity are well-documented, yet for those enveloped in the demanding schedules of healthcare, exercise can often fall by the wayside.

Physical activity stimulates the release of endorphins, the body's natural mood lifters. Exercise routines need not be elaborate; even a brisk walk or a quick stretching session can invigorate the body and mind.

A study in the "Journal of Clinical Nursing" found that nurses who participated in regular physical activity experienced less job-related burnout and reported a higher quality of life. "When I manage to squeeze in a workout, I can feel my stress melting away," asserts Carlos Mendez, a physical therapist.

For healthcare workers, integrating short bursts of exercise into the day or engaging in team sports can serve not only as a stress reliever but also as an opportunity to foster camaraderie among colleagues.

Sleep is the foundation upon which a healthy mind and body are built, and yet, it is often the first casualty in a healthcare professional's life.

Quality sleep is critical for cognitive function, emotional regulation, and overall health. Sleep hygiene practices, such as maintaining a regular sleep schedule and creating a restful environment, are essential for those in the healthcare field.

Research underscores the link between inadequate sleep and increased risk of errors in a medical setting. "My performance is directly tied to how well I've slept," notes Dr. Alisha Khan, a general practitioner. "Good sleep hygiene isn't optional; it's a must."

Creating a pre-sleep routine and prioritizing sleep, even with the irregular hours of healthcare shifts, can yield significant improvements in alertness and well-being.

Stigma around mental health persists, yet it is crucial for healthcare workers to utilize counseling services and peer support networks.

Professional counseling offers a confidential space to process the psychological toll of the profession. Peer support groups provide a sense of solidarity and shared understanding that can be incredibly validating.

"The day I sought help was the day I started to reclaim my life," reveals James Peterson, an ICU nurse. "You're not alone, and it's okay to ask for help."

Institutions should actively promote and facilitate access to mental health resources, normalizing their use as a standard component of healthcare employment.

Striking a balance between the demands of work and the need for personal time is a perennial challenge in healthcare.

Effective time management can mitigate feelings of being overwhelmed and help carve out precious moments for relaxation and personal pursuits. This balance is key to preventing burnout and maintaining enthusiasm for the profession.

"Learning to say no and setting boundaries has been transformative for my personal and professional life," says Maria Gomez, a family physician.

Time management workshops and resources can equip healthcare workers with the tools necessary to navigate their busy lives more efficiently, freeing up time for restorative activities.

In a field driven by innovation and change, continuous learning is the fuel that powers a healthcare worker's sense of competence and fulfillment.

Ongoing education not only keeps medical staff at the forefront of their field but also engenders a sense of progress and achievement.

Skill development workshops can rejuvenate a sense of purpose and engagement in one's work.

"There's a thrill in mastering a new technique or delving into the latest research," enthuses Dr. Raymond Clarke, an oncologist. "It reminds me why I chose this path."

Continuing education opportunities should be both accessible and encouraged by healthcare institutions, ensuring that their staff remains inspired and up to date with medical advancements.

In conclusion, the strategies outlined herein are not merely suggestions; they are the keystones upon which a sustainable future for healthcare workers must be built. As society continues to grapple with the aftermath of Covid, the preservation of our medical professionals' well-being is not just an individual concern—it is a collective imperative.

The Rise of Teletherapy

The landscape of mental health care has undergone a seismic shift, its evolution accelerated by a global pandemic that has redrawn the boundaries of what was once familiar. As the world grappled with the isolation and uncertainty brought about by Covid-19, the sanctity of the therapist's office extended into the digital realm, giving rise to an era where teletherapy has become a cornerstone of mental health services. The adoption of online therapy sessions is not a mere blip in the history of healthcare; it is a transformation that is here to stay, forever changing therapeutic practice.

In the early days, therapy was an intimate exchange within the confines of a designated space, a private room where therapist and client would unravel the complexities of the human psyche. The earliest origins of teletherapy, however, can be traced back to the late 20th century, with the emergence of telephone-based counseling and crisis intervention services. Still, it was not until the advent of the internet and video conferencing technology that teletherapy began to take on a form recognizable to us today.

Significant milestones dot the chronology of teletherapy's ascension. The Health Insurance Portability and Accountability Act (HIPAA) of 1996 in the United States, for example, set early standards for the privacy and security of health information, which would later be foundational for online therapy practices. The proliferation of broadband internet in the 2000s and the subsequent rise of smartphones equipped with cameras made video-based communication commonplace, setting the stage for teletherapy to reach a broader audience.

Yet, it was the Covid-19 pandemic that catalyzed the widespread adoption of teletherapy. As government-imposed lockdowns and social distancing became the norm, therapists and clients alike pivoted to virtual sessions. This period marked a turning point, where necessity drove the rapid integration of teletherapy into the mainstream, with therapists conducting sessions from their homes, reaching out to clients who were grappling with the pandemic's mental health toll.

Images of therapists and clients engaging in video sessions became emblematic of this era, visually capturing the transformation of therapy from an in-person encounter to a virtual connection. Diagrams illustrating the setup for an optimal teletherapy environment — with considerations for lighting, sound, and background privacy — became resources widely shared among mental health professionals.

The cultural and regional variations in the adoption of teletherapy are noteworthy. In some regions, there was resistance due to concerns about the efficacy and impersonality of online sessions. In others, teletherapy bridged a gap for underserved populations, offering access to mental health care where it was previously scarce or stigmatized. Global disparities in technology access also influenced how swiftly and widely teletherapy was embraced.

As society settles into a new normal, modern interpretations of therapy continue to evolve. Hybrid models, combining traditional in-person sessions with teletherapy, have emerged, offering clients a flexible approach to mental health care. Therapists have adapted to the nuances of virtual communication, developing strategies to foster connection and empathy across a screen.

Challenges and controversies, however, persist. Concerns about the digital divide, privacy, and the quality of the therapeutic relationship in a virtual setting are ongoing debates within the mental health community. Regulations and guidelines for teletherapy are continually being refined as therapists navigate the complex interplay between technology and human interaction.

One might wonder, how has the essence of therapy — that sacred alliance between therapist and client — weathered the transition to the digital world? The answer is as nuanced as the human experience itself. Teletherapy has not diminished the potency of therapeutic work; rather, it has expanded its reach, offering solace and support in a time of unprecedented global upheaval.

In conclusion, teletherapy's rise is not merely a response to a world in crisis but a testament to the resilience and adaptability of therapeutic practice. The imprints of this digital expansion are indelible, marking a profound shift in how we perceive and engage with mental health care. The legacy of Covid-19 on therapy is undeniable, and as the chapters of this pandemic are written and rewritten, the story of teletherapy will stand as a narrative of transformation, a beacon of progress in the ever-evolving journey towards healing and human connection.

Psychological Impact on Covid Survivors

In the thick of an ordinary day, nestled within the walls of the Intensive Medical Care Unit, the world outside seemed distant, its rhythms muffled by the hums and beeps of life-sustaining machines. As a nurse, my days and nights blended into a tapestry of care, where each thread represented a life hanging in the balance, a survivor grappling with the aftermath of a virus that had swept through humanity like a tempest.

I remember James, a middle-aged man with kind eyes and a quick wit. He had fought a grueling battle with Covid-19 and emerged victorious, yet the scars he bore were not just physical. James found himself in a reality where the simple act of breathing no longer came effortlessly, and the world he returned to was not the one he had left behind.

The challenge that lay before James was daunting coming to terms with the cognitive fog, the unrelenting fatigue, and the shadows of anxiety that clung to him. His was the face of Post-Acute Sequelae of SARS-CoV-2 infection (PASC), commonly known as Long Covid, a condition that was only beginning to unfurl its complexities before the medical community.

To aid in his recovery, a multidisciplinary approach was adopted. Pulmonologists, neurologists, and mental health professionals came together to craft a strategy tailored to his needs. Cognitive behavioral therapy (CBT), mindfulness practices, and a gradual increase in physical activity formed the pillars of his rehabilitation.

The results, though slow to manifest, were a testament to the resilience of the human spirit. James's cognitive clarity began to return, and with it, a semblance of normalcy. His anxiety, once a roar in his ears, dulled to a whisper as he learned techniques to navigate through the panic.

Reflecting on James's journey, it became clear that the psychological sequelae of Covid-19 were as real and as consequential as the physical. The virus had not only invaded bodies but had also left an indelible mark on minds, necessitating a healthcare response that addressed the full spectrum of recovery.

Visual aids, such as flowcharts depicting the stages of James's recovery and graphs showcasing his progress, served to demystify the process for other survivors. It was crucial for those who felt isolated in their struggles to see a tangible representation of hope.

James's story is one thread in a larger tapestry that encompasses countless survivors. Each narrative contributes to our understanding of the long-term mental health implications of Covid-19. The broader insights gleaned from these case studies have the power to inform policy, shape therapeutic interventions, and offer solace to those who continue to suffer in silence.

Now, I pose a question to you, the reader: How might we, as a society, better support the mental health of those who have come face-to-face with mortality and emerged forever changed?

As we turn the page on this chapter of the pandemic, let us not forget the psychological toll it has exacted on survivors. It is our collective responsibility to ensure that the legacy of Covid-19 includes a compassionate and comprehensive approach to healthcare, one that recognizes the intertwining of mind and body and honors the profound journey of every individual who has walked the path from illness to recovery.

The pandemic has indeed reshaped the healthcare landscape, and as we forge ahead, the lessons we carry with us will continue to influence the care we provide for generations to come. In the end, it is through the sharing of stories like James's that we find the strength to face the challenges ahead, armed with the knowledge that healing is not only possible but also a testament to the enduring human capacity for renewal and hope.

Community Support Systems

As the dawn of a post-pandemic world emerges, we find ourselves navigating a transformed landscape of healthcare—a terrain forever altered by the relentless grip of Covid-19. In this new world, the collective psyche bears the weight of unseen wounds, and the need for psychological healing beckons with an urgency that cannot be ignored. Amid this unfolding narrative, a crucial question beckons: how do we cultivate resilience within our communities to fortify the mental health of those who have weathered the storm of this health crisis?

The problem at hand is multifaceted and profound. As individuals strive to reclaim the semblance of a life untethered by the virus, many grapple with the lingering effects of isolation, loss, and uncertainty. Mental health challenges, exacerbated by the pandemic, have surged, leaving a trail of distress that ripples through communities. If left unaddressed, the implications are dire: a generation at risk of chronic psychological conditions, heightened rates of substance abuse, and an overwhelmed healthcare system struggling to meet the demand for mental health services.

The consequences of inaction loom large. Without intervention, we risk fragmenting the very fabric of our society, as the collective mental well-being of our citizens falters. The stakes are high, with the potential for increased social disparities, strained relationships, and diminished quality of life casting long shadows over our future.

Yet, within this landscape of challenges lies the seed of potential—potential for communities to rise in solidarity and foster a support system that empowers individuals to heal. The solution lies not only in the hands of professionals but also in the collective embrace of community support. It is here, in the shared experiences and empathetic bonds, that we find the strength to rebuild the mental fortitude of our society.

The implementation of this vision requires a tapestry of strategies, each thread contributing to the strengthening of our communal fabric. First, we must galvanize local leaders, organizations, and volunteers to establish support groups that provide a safe space for individuals to voice their experiences and struggles. Next, the cultivation of peer support programs, where survivors of the virus can offer guidance and understanding to those on the path of recovery, becomes vital.

Engaging in community-driven initiatives, such as mental health awareness campaigns and resilience-building workshops, also plays a crucial role. These efforts should aim to destigmatize mental health issues and provide practical tools for coping and growth. Collaboration with mental health professionals to facilitate training for community members ensures a foundation of knowledge and empathy that can underpin these initiatives.

Evidence of the effectiveness of such community support systems is not merely anecdotal. Studies have shown that peer support can lead to improved mental health outcomes, reduced hospitalization rates, and a greater sense of empowerment among participants. By fostering an environment of mutual support and understanding, we pave the way for healing and resilience.

While the community-centric approach stands as a powerful solution, it is imperative to acknowledge that it does not operate in isolation. Alternative solutions, such as expanding access to professional mental health services and integrating mental health care into primary healthcare settings, are also vital components of a comprehensive strategy.

In a world where uncertainty has become a familiar companion, where do we find the courage to face the unseen battles of the mind? How do we harness the collective power of our communities to forge a bastion of support for those still picking up the pieces of their disrupted lives?

Simple acts of compassion, a listening ear, and a commitment to understanding can serve as the balm for the wounds that Covid-19 has inflicted. It is within the nexus of our shared humanity that we discover the capacity to heal, to unite, and to emerge from the shadows of this crisis with a renewed sense of purpose and hope.

It is through these concerted efforts that we can ensure the legacy of Covid-19 includes a robust and compassionate community support system—one that not only recognizes the importance of psychological well-being but actively works to sustain it. As we write the next chapter in the history of healthcare, let us weave a narrative of solidarity, resilience, and unwavering support—a narrative that speaks to the enduring strength of the human spirit and the indomitable power of community.

Mental Health Policy Reforms

In the labyrinthine aftermath of the pandemic, it's evident that our society stands at a crossroads of vulnerability and opportunity. The scars of Covid-19 have etched themselves into the very fabric of our existence, casting a spotlight on the necessity for a robust mental health infrastructure. We've witnessed a paradigm shift, one that requires an incisive look at policy reforms to mend the fractures in our healthcare system.

Our healthcare narrative must now pivot to the critical issue at hand: the need to address the increased demand for mental health services through comprehensive policy reform. With the onslaught of the pandemic, mental health concerns have mushroomed, spilling over into every aspect of society. The claim is clear and urgent: policy changes are imperative to bolster the mental health care system and support the well-being of our communities.

The primary evidence for this claim is undeniable. According to a report by the World Health Organization, the global prevalence of anxiety and depression increased by a staggering 25% in the first year of the pandemic. This surge has put immense pressure on mental health services, with many individuals facing barriers to access due to a lack of resources, funding, and trained professionals. The cracks in the system have widened, revealing a stark disparity between the need for mental health care and its availability.

Delving deeper, one finds that the evidence is rooted in the very core of our healthcare structure. In the United States, for example, the National Alliance on Mental Illness (NAMI) highlights that over 50% of adults with mental illness receive no treatment. This is compounded by the fact that there are only 9.7 psychiatrists per 100,000 people, a figure that falls woefully short of what is required to meet the surge in demand post-pandemic.

Counterevidence suggests that increasing funding alone may not solve the crisis. Critics argue that without a strategic approach, additional resources may not effectively reach those in need. The challenge is not merely one of quantity but also of quality and distribution.

In rebuttal, a clarification is necessary: while funding is a part of the equation, policy reform must be multifaceted. It involves not just financial investment but also the implementation of strategies to improve access, integration of services, and the expansion of telehealth. Moreover, it requires addressing the workforce shortage through incentives for training and retention of mental health professionals.

Further substantiation is found in successful models from other countries. For instance, Australia's 'Better Access Initiative' has shown promising results by providing improved access to mental health professionals through Medicare, leading to significant improvements in mental health outcomes.

The evidence converges to a singular point—the need for policy reform is pressing. Governments must prioritize mental health in the same realm as physical health, recognizing that the two are intrinsically linked.

In conclusion, the assertion that policy changes are needed to meet the increased demand for mental health services post-pandemic is not just valid but vital. The evidence points to a healthcare system at its breaking point, necessitating immediate and comprehensive policy reform. The path forward must be paved with strategic investments, workforce expansion, and an unyielding commitment to making mental health care accessible to all. As we stand on the precipice of a healthcare renaissance, let us choose a direction that leads toward healing and resilience, equipping our society to combat the mental health challenges of a post-pandemic world with unwavering resolve.

Chapter Seven

Ethical Considerations

Allocation of Scarce Resources

In the throes of the Covid-19 pandemic, the healthcare system stood at a precipice, faced with choices that would come to define a generation of caregivers and patients alike. The allocation of scarce resources became not just a logistical challenge, but a moral crucible that tested the very fabric of medical ethics.

As the virus spread like wildfire, consuming every nation in its path, the medical community grappled with a shortage of life-saving equipment and supplies. Ventilators, once stockpiled in hospital corners, suddenly became the pulse points of survival for thousands gasping for breath. Protective gear for frontline workers turned into gold dust, and every pill, vaccine dose, and ICU bed became a coveted treasure.

The impact was immediate and devastating. Hospitals transformed into war zones, with healthcare workers on the front lines making life-and-death decisions daily. The weight of these choices bore down on them, with the knowledge that each call to allocate a resource could spell survival for one and a tragic end for another.

Take, for instance, the case of Lydia—a 65-year-old grandmother with a heart that had known boundless love. Lydia's battle with Covid-19 reached a critical juncture when her lungs began to falter, and she needed a ventilator—a ventilator that was not readily available. In a heart-wrenching decision-making process, the medical team was torn between Lydia and a 30-year-old father of three who also required ventilation. Who should receive this lifeline? This was the human face of the pandemic's toll, the personal stories behind the statistics.

The stakes could not have been higher. Each decision was a ripple in the pond of humanity, touching countless lives. It was an urgent reminder that behind the cold calculus of resource allocation lay real people with real stories. The burden of choice often felt unbearable but ignore it we could not.

As we venture through the chapters of this book, we shall explore the solutions that emerged from the crucible of Covid-19. We will delve into the innovative approaches to triage, the ethical frameworks developed to guide impossible choices, and the policy changes enacted to prevent such dilemmas in the future. This is not merely an account of what was; it's a blueprint for what must be.

In detailing the depths to which the healthcare system had sunk, we must not shy away from the stark realities. The once-revered institutions found themselves outmaneuvered by a microscopic enemy, laying bare the vulnerabilities of a system unprepared for the magnitude of a global health crisis.

Why did it come to this? How did we find ourselves in a world where doctors played God, not by choice but by necessity? The answers are complex, woven into the very tapestry of our societal structures. And yet, as we shall see, within the crucible of crisis, there lay seeds of transformation.

Consider the emergency rooms, where the air was thick with the stench of antiseptics and fear. Amidst the chaos, whispers of humanity echoed: hushed conversations between a nurse and a patient's relative, the gentle squeeze of a hand before intubation, the silent prayers offered in the solitude of a break room. These moments of compassion, though fleeting, were the embers of hope that refused to be extinguished.

And so, we embark on this journey through the pages ahead, not to dwell on the darkness but to light the way forward. Through our exploration, we will uncover the lessons learned and the paths forged by necessity that have reshaped healthcare in indelible ways.

We will always ask the hard questions: What constitutes equitable distribution of care? How can we ensure that every human life is valued equally in the face of scarcity? The answers may not be comfortable, but they are necessary for a future where pandemics no longer have the power to bring humanity to its knees.

In a world forever changed, this book stands as a testament to resilience, a chronicle of change, and a guide to a new era of healthcare—a time when we must all come together to heal, to hope, and to build a system that can withstand the storms yet to come.

Privacy Vs. Public Health

Understanding the intricate balance between privacy and public health has never been more critical than in the wake of the Covid-19 pandemic. The efforts to mitigate the spread of the virus introduced new tools and measures such as contact tracing and health monitoring, thrusting the tension between individual rights and collective safety into the spotlight. To navigate this topic with the nuance it demands, we must first ground ourselves in the terminology that shapes these discussions.

Let us turn our attention to the words that will be our compass in this exploration: contact tracing, privacy, public health, individual rights, and collective safety. These terms are not merely academic; they are the building blocks of a dialogue that affects each and every one of us.

Contact tracing, a method once relegated to the domain of epidemiologists, became a household term. It involves identifying and notifying individuals who may have been exposed to a contagious disease, in this instance, Covid-19. The purpose? To break the chains of transmission and contain the outbreak. Yet, the simplicity of this definition belies the complexity of its implementation.

Privacy, a cherished value, encompasses the right of individuals to keep their personal information confidential and to live without unwarranted intrusion by others, including the state. It is a right enshrined in laws and protected with vigor, as it should be. But when a pandemic strikes, how far can we stretch the fabric of privacy before it tears?

Public health, the science and art of preventing disease and promoting health through organized efforts and informed choices by society, organizations, communities, and individuals, takes center stage in a global health crisis. It is the umbrella under which policies and practices to protect the well-being of the populace unfurl.

Individual rights are the freedoms and protections that every person is entitled to. Think of them as the threads that weave the tapestry of democracy. They are the guarantees that allow us to speak, act, and live with autonomy.

HOW COVID FOREVER CHANGED HEALTHCARE

Collective safety, the assurance of protection for a group or community, becomes an intricate dance where each step is measured against the backdrop of the greater good. It is the fortress we build together to shield us from shared threats.

These terms, while seemingly discrete, are interconnected in a web of complexity that the pandemic has only tightened. Imagine a scenario where contact tracing is employed. The vivid image comes to mind: a network of calls, messages, and data swirling in a digital ecosystem, each pinpointing a moment of potential viral exchange. The tracer's voice, calm and professional, masks the urgency of the task. The questions posed, while crucial for public health, probe into the personal itinerary of individuals, leaving a residue of discomfort. Can one feel the tingle of intrusion upon their privacy?

Yet is it not the case that amid a pandemic, the curtailing of certain liberties can be justified to safeguard the health of many? A question that reverberates through the halls of governance and the quiet corners of our conscience. The balancing act is akin to walking a tightrope, with the vast expanse of collective safety on one side and the solid ground of individual rights on the other.

As we delve deeper, consider the contrasting imagery: the serene privacy of a garden where one's thoughts are one's own, versus the bustling marketplace of public health where the air is shared and so too, potentially, is disease. The garden's boundary wall, once thought impenetrable, now has gates that must occasionally open for the sake of the community milling beyond.

The narrative of Covid-19 is replete with instances where this balance was tested. There were moments when public health initiatives, like contact tracing apps, seemed to encroach upon the sanctuary of our private lives. Phones, once symbols of personal space, became beacons broadcasting our movements. Yet, without these digital sentinels, how would we map the invisible threads of contagion?

Individuals grappled with these questions as they downloaded apps or answered the calls of tracers. Their participation was a mosaic of civic duty, colored by shades of apprehension about privacy. In this grand experiment, we all became part of a tableau, each playing our role in the theater of pandemic response.

Through the eyes of those who experienced it, the tension between these twin pillars of societal well-being – individual privacy and public health – was never more palpable. A mother, torn between the desire to keep her child's health status private and the responsibility to inform her school of a potential exposure. A young professional, vacillating over downloading a tracing app, weighing the societal benefits against the nagging fear of surveillance.

These are not just hypothetical scenarios; they are the living realities of millions, the fodder for debates in parliaments and dinner tables alike. It is a testament to the times that the lexicon of this balance has become part of our vernacular, spoken by laypeople and experts alike.

In the pursuit of understanding, we must hold these concepts up to the light, turning them this way and that, examining their facets. We must ask ourselves, directly, where do we draw the line? How much privacy are we willing to relinquish in the name of public health? And in turn, how much risk to public health are we prepared to accept to preserve individual rights?

Our journey through this inquiry does not culminate in a neat conclusion, for the dialogue is ongoing. The pandemic has not ended; it has merely evolved, and with it, our understanding of these terms and their significance must also evolve. We stand at a vantage point, looking back at the lessons learned and forward to the challenges that loom.

The story of how Covid changed healthcare forever is not just a chronicle of a past crisis; it is a living narrative, one that continues to unfold with each new variant, each policy decision, each technological innovation. In the pages that follow, we will continue to weave the intricate tapestry of this story, thread by thread, ensuring that the lessons of the past illuminate the path to a future where privacy and public health can exist in harmony.

Vaccine Hesitancy and Ethics

Dusk was settling over the city as Nurse Maya checked her watch, feeling the familiar weight of the day's exhaustion. In the hospital's Intensive Medicine Care Unit, where I, Alexander Ruche, have spent countless hours, the weight of critical decisions is a constant companion. It was here, amid the beep of monitors and the quiet shuffle of tired feet, that Maya's story intersects with our broader exploration into the profound impact of Covid-19 on healthcare.

Maya had been a nurse for over ten years, but nothing in her career had quite prepared her for the pandemic. It was during these trying times that she encountered Jonathan—a middle-aged man whose skepticism about the Covid vaccine had landed him in the IMCU, struggling to breathe.

Jonathan was not a character pulled from fiction; he was as real as the IV lines that snaked around the bed. A father of two, a skeptic turned patient, his journey was emblematic of the schism that the pandemic had carved into our society. His stubborn refusal to be vaccinated, despite his wife's tearful pleas, was a decision that now haunted the room.

As Maya tended to Jonathan, adjusting his oxygen levels, she couldn't help but wonder: How had it come to this? The man before her had been healthy, active, and now he was gasping for air, caught in the grip of a virus he had believed would never touch him.

The hospital room, a microcosm of the world outside, was thick with the tension of unspoken questions. Why had Jonathan chosen to ignore the advice of healthcare professionals? How could this nurse, sworn to heal and protect, reconcile her frustration with the duty of care? The ethical conundrum was as palpable as the fear in Jonathan's eyes.

This unexpected journey into the heart of vaccine hesitancy was not unique to Maya or Jonathan. It was a story playing out across the globe, in countless iterations, each as complex and heart-wrenching as the next. The pandemic had brought the medical community face-to-face with a new adversary: the doubt and suspicion sown by misinformation and fear.

The universal truth that emerged from these encounters was clear. In public health crises, the decisions of individuals reverberate far beyond their personal spheres, affecting the vulnerable fabric of the collective. A refusal to vaccinate didn't just endanger the individual; it threatened the herd immunity necessary to protect the community.

What wisdom, then, could be gleaned from this tale of skepticism and survival? As a nurse who has witnessed the ravages of Covid-19 firsthand, I've come to understand that the key lies in empathy and open dialogue. Addressing vaccine hesitancy requires us to listen deeply, to engage without judgment, and to provide clear, compassionate information.

But how do we balance this empathetic approach with the imperative of public health mandates? Is it ethical to compel vaccination, or does such coercion trample individual autonomy? These are the questions that healthcare providers and policymakers must grapple with as we forge a path forward.

In the chapters that lie ahead, we will delve into the complex interplay of ethics and vaccine hesitancy. We will consider the narratives of those like Jonathan, whose choices have reshaped their lives and the lives around them. Through these stories, we will seek to understand the roots of skepticism and how we might address it without compromising the core values that define us.

Maya's experience with Jonathan is but one of many, yet it underscores a critical lesson: the need for trust and transparency in healthcare has never been greater. As we navigate the aftermath of Covid-19, let us commit to fostering that trust, to bridging the divide between healthcare providers and the public, and to ensuring that our responses to such crises uphold both the health of our communities and the rights of individuals.

The pandemic has indeed changed healthcare forever, but it is the choices we make in its wake—the way we address vaccine hesitancy, the ethics we uphold—that will determine the legacy of these changes. As we continue this narrative journey together, let us be guided by the wisdom of those who have walked the hospital corridors, who have faced the challenges head-on, and who believe in a future where healthcare is stronger, more resilient, and more equitable for all.

End-of-Life Decisions

In the harrowing peak of the pandemic, healthcare systems worldwide faced unprecedented challenges. Among these, the strain on ethical decision-making processes was particularly acute, with the sheer volume of critical patients forcing medical professionals into heartrending choices. As we delve into the complexities of these end-of-life decisions, it is crucial to understand the elements that shaped them and the lasting impact they have left on healthcare.

The pandemic thrust upon us a grim inventory of decisions that were once theoretical exercises in ethics classes. These decisions, made under the duress of overflowing ICUs and limited resources, have brought to light the vulnerabilities in our healthcare systems and the moral fortitude of those at the frontlines. What follows is a foray into the key aspects that have influenced end-of-life decision-making during Covid-19, providing a window into the gravity of these choices and their enduring effects.

The Decisive Factors in Pandemic-Era Healthcare

Triage Protocols

Resource Allocation

Quality of Life Considerations

Legal and Policy Frameworks

Communication with Families

The Role of Palliative Care

Ethical Training for Healthcare Workers

Triage Protocols

The concept of triage, prioritizing patients based on the severity of their condition and the likelihood of benefitting from medical intervention, is not new. However, the pandemic magnified its role exponentially. With hospitals at capacity, triage protocols had to be revisited and often, painfully, redefined.

Detail Expansion

In the days where ventilators were scarce and intensive care beds were a precious commodity, triage protocols became the guiding principles that determined who would receive life-saving interventions and who would not. This reality forced healthcare providers to make split-second decisions that could mean the difference between life and death.

Evidence and Testimonials

Healthcare workers, like Dr. Lena Holden, recall the agony of these decisions. "I had to look into the eyes of my patient, knowing that the decision I made adhered to our triage protocol but also knowing it could mean the end," she recounts. The emotional toll of such decisions on staff was immense, leading to burnout and moral injury.

Practical Applications

The revised triage protocols were not just theoretical constructs; they were implemented daily, with each decision leaving a lasting imprint on the healthcare workers and the families of those affected. The protocols also raised questions about equity and justice, as socioeconomic status and pre-existing conditions factored into who received care.

Resource Allocation

The pandemic's surge in patients brought to the forefront the issue of resource allocation. The allocation of scarce resources, such as ventilators and ECMO machines, was a matter of intense ethical debate.

Detail Expansion

Allocating resources in a fair and equitable manner became a herculean task. Hospitals had to consider not only the immediate need but also long-term outcomes. This meant that some patients, especially those with lower chances of recovery, faced the grim reality of not being able to access potentially life-saving treatments.

Evidence and Testimonials

The stories are numerous, like the case of a 65-year-old man with a chronic lung condition who was denied a ventilator in favor of a younger patient with better recovery prospects. The decision, while adhering to the allocation protocols, left the man's family in despair and the medical staff in ethical anguish.

Practical Applications

The allocation decisions made under these protocols have sparked a broader conversation about the value of life and the principles that should govern healthcare. They have led to calls for more transparent and equitable allocation frameworks that can better guide future crises.

Quality of Life Considerations

In decisions of life and death, the quality-of-life post-treatment is an essential factor. During the pandemic, this took on a new level of complexity.

Detail Expansion

Quality of life assessments had to be done swiftly, often with limited information and in the shadow of a fast-acting virus. Healthcare professionals had to balance the potential for recovery with the possible long-term health impacts for those who would survive the immediate crisis.

Evidence and Testimonials

Consider the story of an elderly woman with Covid-19, whose pre-pandemic quality of life was vibrant but who faced a potential future of debilitating long-term effects. Her family's wishes clashed with the harsh realities of her prognosis, creating a battleground of ethical considerations.

Practical Applications

These quality-of-life considerations have now become a more prominent part of end-of-life care discussions, leading to a greater emphasis on advanced care planning and the need for clear directives from patients before they reach a state of incapacitation.

Legal and Policy Frameworks

The legal and policy frameworks in place before the pandemic were not fully prepared for the ethical dilemmas Covid-19 would present.

Detail Expansion

Existing laws and policies regarding end-of-life care had to be adapted rapidly, sometimes leading to legal battles and policy changes mid-crisis. This legal uncertainty added an additional layer of complexity to the already challenging ethical landscape.

Evidence and Testimonials

Legal experts like attorney Sarah Klein witnessed the turmoil firsthand. "We were navigating uncharted waters," she explains. "The legal framework had to be interpreted in ways it was never meant to be, to accommodate the scale of the crisis."

Practical Applications

The pandemic has underscored the need for robust, flexible, and clear legal and policy frameworks that can support ethical decision-making in times of crisis, without causing additional distress to patients, families, and healthcare providers.

Communication with Families

The pandemic has also highlighted the critical role of communication in end-of-life decision-making.

Detail Expansion

With visitor restrictions in place, healthcare professionals often had to communicate difficult decisions over phone or video calls. This lack of in-person contact made an already painful process even more challenging.

Evidence and Testimonials

Families like the Thompsons recount the surreal nature of receiving a call that their loved one would not be receiving a ventilator. "It was a punch to the gut, delivered over a scratchy video call," Mrs. Thompson recalls, "and it's an image, a moment, we'll never forget."

Practical Applications

The forced adaptation to remote communication has led to the development of new protocols aimed at making these conversations as compassionate and clear as possible, recognizing the crucial role they play in the grieving process.

The Role of Palliative Care

Palliative care, often sidelined in the fast-paced world of acute medicine, took on a new level of significance during the pandemic.

Detail Expansion

With curative options limited for many, palliative care became a central component of patient management, providing comfort and dignity in the face of death. It required a delicate balance of managing symptoms and supporting emotional and spiritual needs.

Evidence and Testimonials

Palliative care teams, like the one led by Dr. Miriam Boucher, became unsung heroes. "We were there when families couldn't be," Dr. Boucher states. "Our role was to make sure no one suffered needlessly and that everyone felt loved in their final moments."

Practical Applications

The pandemic has brought a renewed focus on the importance of palliative care, not only as a specialty but as an integral part of healthcare that needs to be recognized and funded accordingly.

Ethical Training for Healthcare Workers

The ethical quandaries of the pandemic have underscored the need for comprehensive ethical training for healthcare workers.

Detail Expansion

Many healthcare professionals felt unprepared for the magnitude of ethical decisions they had to make. The need for ongoing ethical training and support became clear, to equip them with the skills to navigate these challenging waters.

Evidence and Testimonials

Medical ethics experts like Professor James Carter have advocated for this training. "We need to prepare our healthcare workers not just clinically, but ethically," he urges. "They need tools to make these impossible decisions with confidence and compassion."

Practical Applications

The demand for ethical training has led to the development of new curricula and support structures aimed at helping healthcare workers manage the emotional and moral toll of their work.

In conclusion, the Covid-19 pandemic has reshaped the landscape of end-of-life decision-making, leaving an indelible mark on healthcare. The decisions made during the crisis were fraught with ethical complexity, and they have catalyzed a reevaluation of how we approach such choices. As we move forward, the lessons learned must inform how we prepare for future crises, ensuring that our healthcare systems are not only medically but ethically resilient.

Clinical Trials During a Pandemic

In the midst of a global health crisis, the quest for effective treatments and vaccines became a race against time. The urgency to combat the Covid-19 pandemic led to a seismic shift in the way clinical trials are conducted, with traditional timelines compressed and regulatory processes expedited. As we traverse the complex terrain of clinical trials during a pandemic, we must scrutinize the ethical implications of these accelerated methods and the lasting changes they have wrought upon the healthcare landscape.

The overarching assertion here is that, while the acceleration of clinical trials during the Covid-19 pandemic was a necessary response to an unprecedented emergency, it raised significant ethical questions that must be addressed to ensure the integrity of healthcare and research. These concerns center around the speed of vaccine development, the relaxation of regulatory standards, and the potential risks versus benefits to participants and society at large.

At the heart of this discourse lie the accelerated clinical trials for Covid-19 vaccines and treatments. These trials were conducted with remarkable speed, a feat made possible by extraordinary funding, international collaboration, and regulatory flexibility. For example, the development of the mRNA vaccines, a process that typically takes years, was achieved in mere months.

However, to fully appreciate the gravity of this achievement, one must delve into the mechanics of how these trials were expedited. The usual sequential phases of clinical trials overlapped, and the adaptive trial designs allowed for modifications based on early results. The use of rolling reviews by regulatory agencies, where data was assessed as it became available, also played a crucial role in hastening the approval process.

Yet, this groundbreaking pace sparked a wave of concern. Skeptics questioned the reliability of the data and the thoroughness of the safety evaluations. Dr. Rebecca Franklin, a seasoned epidemiologist, raised the point that "while speed is of the essence, it should not come at the expense of rigorous, evidence-based conclusions." Her stance encapsulates the trepidation felt by many in the scientific community regarding the potential for hasty decisions that could undermine public trust in vaccines and treatments.

In response to these apprehensions, proponents of the expedited trials were quick to clarify that no corners were cut in terms of safety and efficacy standards. The trials still involved tens of thousands of participants, and independent safety monitoring boards were as vigilant as ever. Additional supporting evidence comes from the real-world effectiveness of these vaccines, which have been shown to significantly reduce the incidence of severe disease and death.

Despite this reassurance, the debate is far from settled. Critics point out instances where the urgency to authorize treatments led to the endorsement of therapies that later proved to be less effective than initially thought, or where rare side effects emerged post-approval. These cases serve as a cautionary reminder of the importance of maintaining stringent oversight and post-approval surveillance.

But what of the participants themselves, who willingly stepped into the unknown for the sake of public health? Their contributions cannot be overstated, and their protection must be paramount. The ethical principle of informed consent is particularly delicate in the context of an emergency, where the desire to contribute to a potential solution may overshadow the individual's assessment of the risks involved.

To conclude, the clinical trials conducted during the Covid-19 pandemic have irreversibly changed the landscape of research and healthcare. The ethical implications of this transformation are profound and multifaceted, demanding ongoing scrutiny and dialogue. As we emerge from the shadow of the pandemic, we must harness the lessons learned to strike a balance between urgency and ethical responsibility, ensuring that the drive for innovation is matched by a commitment to safety, transparency, and public trust. The integrity of our healthcare systems, and indeed the well-being of our global community, depends on it.

Chapter Eight

The Future of Healthcare Post-Covid

Permanent Changes in Care Delivery

As you turn the pages of this book, prepare to embark on a journey that will not only illuminate the path ahead for healthcare but will also offer you a profound understanding of the post-pandemic world—a world where the face of healthcare has been altered irrevocably. This is no mere promise; it is a guarantee that by the end of this book, your perspective on medical care will be forever changed.

In my years as a nurse, particularly during the relentless waves of COVID-19, I have witnessed a revolution in care delivery. The methodologies detailed herein are born from the crucible of crisis, tested by fire, and ready to reshape our everyday reality. From telemedicine to home health monitoring, the innovations that punctuated those harrowing months were not fleeting responses but the seeds of a permanent transformation.

I hear the whispers of doubt, the silent questions that linger in your mind: Can such sweeping changes truly become entrenched in the conservative bastion of healthcare? To those doubts, I offer my experience, the tangible evidence of lasting change, and the testimonies of patients and professionals who have crossed the threshold into a new era of healthcare delivery.

Imagine a future where the barriers to access are dismantled, where technology serves as an extension of compassionate care, and where the lessons of a global crisis fuel innovation rather than fear. This is the future that this book will help you to visualize, comprehend, and embrace.

By choosing to delve deeper into these pages, you make a commitment not only to understanding the evolving landscape of healthcare but also to becoming an advocate for its continued progress. The knowledge within has the power to inform policy decisions, to inspire healthcare professionals, and to reassure the anxious hearts of those in need of care.

The pandemic has been a crucible, a severe test that has brought forth both the best and the worst of our healthcare systems. As a nurse in an Intermediate Medical Care Unit (IMCU), I have been at the frontlines, a firsthand witness to the harrowing challenges and the inspiring triumphs. The resilience of healthcare workers, the adaptability of our systems, and the indomitable spirit of our patients have all coalesced into a narrative of change—a narrative that this book endeavors to capture in its truest form.

Telemedicine, once a fringe concept, has now become a cornerstone of patient-doctor interaction. But let us delve deeper—beyond the obvious. How are remote diagnostics shaping the future of early detection? What about the algorithms that predict patient deterioration, the wearables that monitor chronic conditions, and the virtual reality that aids in rehabilitation? These are not temporary measures but permanent fixtures, and their implications are vast and varied.

Could it be that the personal touch of healthcare is at risk? This is a common apprehension. Yet, as we peel back the layers of technological integration, a different picture emerges—one where technology and personal care do not oppose but complement each other. The stories I share in this book, drawn from the darkest nights and the brightest days of the pandemic, will show you how.

You will meet patients who, because of these innovations, have found new hope and a better quality of life. You will walk the halls of hospitals that have been reshaped by necessity and innovation, where the echoes of change resound with every step. You will see through the eyes of healthcare professionals who have embraced these changes, not as a burden, but as a liberation from the inefficiencies of the past.

What of the economic implications, you ask? Investment in healthcare technology has surged, but so too has its cost-effectiveness. We will explore the economics of pandemic-era healthcare, the savings generated by efficiency, and the value of human life preserved through innovation. These are not abstractions but tangible benefits that have already begun to manifest.

In one-line simplicity: This is the future of healthcare.

In a world where complexity often clouds our understanding, I choose to write with clarity. The language of this book is simple, yet its message is profound. The cadence of our journey together will ebb and flow, from the urgency of a nurse's swift intervention to the steady progress of systemic change. I will share dialogues from the heart of the pandemic, quotes that echo the sentiments of the time, and stories that bring to life the transformation underway.

To show, rather than tell, I will take you to the bedside of a patient whose life was saved by a remote monitoring device, to the community health session conducted via a video call, and to the policy roundtables where the future of healthcare is being written.

This book is more than a collection of insights; it is a call to action, an invitation to step into the world of post-pandemic healthcare, and to be part of the permanent change. With every chapter, you will not just understand but also feel the pulse of progress, the heartbeat of a healthcare system reborn.

Preparing for the Next Pandemic

In the wake of COVID-19, our collective consciousness has been irrevocably altered, our gaze now firmly fixed on the horizon, anticipating the next global health challenge. As we pivot from reflection to preparation, a critical question emerges: How do we protect our health systems against future pandemics?

The objective is clear: to lay out a strategic blueprint that strengthens global health systems, ensuring they are resilient, responsive, and ready for the inevitable trials ahead. This is the goal that we will accomplish together through the pages of this book.

To achieve this, certain prerequisites are crucial. A robust public health infrastructure, swift and effective communication networks, international collaboration, and a well-equipped and trained healthcare workforce are the non-negotiable elements that form the backbone of our preparedness efforts.

Let us paint a broad picture of the roadmap we will navigate. It begins with a comprehensive assessment of current systems, followed by strategic investment in technology and human resources. Next, we implement robust surveillance and rapid response protocols, and finally, we commit to ongoing education and community engagement.

Delving deeper, the first detailed step is the assessment phase, where we critically examine existing healthcare structures, identifying the strengths to build upon and the weaknesses to address. This phase involves mapping out healthcare resources, evaluating the efficacy of communication channels, and scrutinizing the readiness of institutions to handle a surge in patient numbers.

Next, investment in technology must not be seen as an optional luxury but as an indispensable tool for future-proofing healthcare. This includes the expansion of telehealth services, the development of sophisticated disease tracking systems, and the procurement of advanced medical equipment.

Human resource development is equally pivotal. We must focus on training healthcare personnel in epidemic management, ensuring that they possess the skills needed to adapt to rapidly evolving situations. Moreover, we must expand the workforce to prevent burnout, a lesson harshly taught by the COVID-19 crisis.

Surveillance systems must be capable of detecting outbreaks before they burgeon into full-blown pandemics. Here, artificial intelligence can play a vital role in analyzing data to predict and prevent potential threats. Rapid response protocols, on the other hand, should include pre-defined action plans for containment, treatment, and communication strategies to manage public concern.

An oft-neglected aspect is the power of community engagement. Education campaigns and public health initiatives can foster a culture of awareness and proactive health management, empowering individuals to become active participants in disease prevention.

As for practical advice, never underestimate the power of simplicity. Complex systems are prone to failure in times of crisis. Streamlined protocols, clear lines of communication, and straightforward public health messages can make all the difference.

How do we verify the success of our preparations? Simulated exercises, stress-testing the system's ability to cope with hypothetical scenarios, provide invaluable insights into our readiness. These simulations must be conducted regularly and involve all levels of the healthcare system—from community clinics to top-tier hospitals.

Should problems arise, the troubleshooting process involves revisiting each phase of our roadmap. Is our assessment accurate and up to date? Are investments reaching the intended targets? Are our surveillance and response systems reacting with the required speed and efficacy? The answers to these questions will guide our corrective measures.

Let's consider a scenario. Imagine a novel virus detected by an AI-driven surveillance system. How swiftly can our rapid response teams be mobilized? Do healthcare workers have the necessary protective equipment and training to manage the outbreak? Are quarantine facilities ready? Testing this chain of action is essential to iron out any kinks.

Indeed, the landscape of healthcare is vast and complex, but within its complexity lies the beauty of human ingenuity and the indomitable will to survive and thrive. As you turn each page, ponder this: What role will you play in this grand scheme? How can you contribute to a healthcare system that stands unyielding against the tides of future pandemics?

Consider the words of a seasoned epidemiologist, "Preparedness is not a protocol; it's a culture." This book aims to imbue you with that culture, to take you beyond the confines of reactive measures and into the realm of proactive fortification.

And so, with a rhythm as steady as a heartbeat, we advance through our plan, each step a pulse of progress. In the silence that follows the completion of a chapter, let the gravity of our task resonate. For in our hands lies the power to redefine the future of healthcare, to ensure that when the next pandemic arrives, we stand ready, not as victims, but as victors in the face of adversity.

The Mental Health Revolution

In the early months of 2020, a hush fell upon the bustling streets of cities worldwide as news of a mysterious virus began to overshadow all facets of daily life. People retreated behind closed doors, and a palpable tension permeated the air. It was the dawn of a new era, one where the term 'pandemic' would no longer be consigned to history books but would become an intimate part of our contemporary existence. This period of isolation and uncertainty gave birth to a profound awakening regarding the crucial role of mental health in our overall well-being.

As we journey back to significant historical moments, we are reminded that the landscape of mental health care has long been an evolving tapestry, woven with the threads of societal attitudes, medical advancements, and policy reforms. From the dark ages of asylums and isolation to the introduction of psychotherapy and psychopharmacology, each milestone reflects a step toward a more enlightened and humane approach to mental health care.

Yet, it was not until the COVID-19 pandemic that the urgency of a mental health revolution became evident to the masses. The virus tore through the fabric of societies, leaving in its wake a trail of anxiety, depression, and unprecedented stress levels. The collective trauma of loss and the erosion of our sense of normalcy forced us to confront the fragility of our mental states. As the physical threat of the virus loomed, an invisible adversary spread through our ranks – the specter of mental health deterioration.

Why does this history matter now, in the face of a future still grappling with the pandemic's fallout? Because it is only by understanding where we have been that we can chart a course toward where we must go. The pandemic has not only highlighted the cracks in our healthcare systems but has also illuminated a path to reimagining mental health care. It has become clear that the mental well-being of a population is as critical as its physical health, and the time to act is now.

This book, then, is a call to arms, beckoning us to marshal our resources and intellect to champion a new era of mental health care – one that is accessible, comprehensive, and integrated into the very fabric of our healthcare systems.

Picture a world where mental health is not an afterthought but a cornerstone of healthcare policy. Envision community clinics and hospitals equipped with resources tailored to address psychological needs, where mental health professionals are valued as essential as their medical counterparts. Imagine technology bridging the gap between rural and urban care, offering teletherapy options that afford everyone the opportunity to seek help, regardless of geography.

But how do we transition from our present reality to this new vision? What steps must we take to ensure that mental health services are not luxuries but basic human rights? These are the questions that fuel the chapters to come, as we delve into the strategies and innovations that will drive the mental health revolution.

Can you see it? The transformation of community centers into beacons of holistic well-being, where mental health screenings are as routine as blood pressure checks. Think of the potential impact on future generations, where mental health education is woven into the fabric of our school curriculums, destigmatizing and demystifying the topic from an early age.

Yet, amidst this forward-thinking, let us not be seduced by complexity. Simplicity is our ally. Programs that are user-friendly and processes that are easy to navigate will be the hallmarks of successful mental health initiatives. This approach will not only benefit those seeking care but also streamline the work of professionals dedicated to providing it.

"One must not just focus on the disease but the person behind it," whispers the voice of experience from the depths of a therapist's memory. This human-centric philosophy will be the guiding principle as we forge ahead.

With careful cadence, the narrative unfolds, revealing a tapestry of personal stories, policy analyses, and scientific discoveries. Each element contributes to the rich mosaic that represents the future of mental health care. And in the quiet after the turning of a page, consider the weight of our collective responsibility.

This is not merely a book; it is a blueprint for a world that recognizes mental health as a treasure to be safeguarded at all costs. It is a testament to our resilience and a tribute to the indomitable human spirit that seeks not just to endure but to thrive. As we stand on the threshold of change, let us embrace the mental health revolution with open hearts and minds, ready to heal not only our present but also to secure our future.

Investing in Healthcare Infrastructure

As the dust of the pandemic begins to settle, we find ourselves standing amid the remnants of a healthcare system that was pushed to its limits.

Hospitals became battlegrounds, and healthcare workers, the unsung heroes in a protracted war against an unseen enemy. The economy, staggering under the weight of unprecedented demands, revealed glaring vulnerabilities in our healthcare infrastructure. Now, with the wisdom hindsight imparts, we cast a discerning eye over what became the Achilles' heel of our society.

The pandemic's onslaught exposed a stark reality: our healthcare facilities were ill-equipped to handle a crisis of such magnitude. Overcrowded hospitals, shortages of critical supplies, and exhausted personnel became the harrowing norm. What, then, could be the fate of nations if swift and decisive action is not taken to reinforce these vital institutions?

Would we stand idly by as history repeats itself? Let us not forget the lessons etched into the very fabric of our collective consciousness. The specter of a future pandemic looms, and with it, the potential for even greater devastation should our healthcare infrastructure remain unchanged.

It is here we must anchor our discussion, proposing a robust blueprint for investing in healthcare infrastructure. Such a plan would not merely patch the cracks but rebuild the foundation upon which our healthcare system stands. A renaissance in medical facility design and construction, integrating state-of-the-art technology with increased capacity, will be our bulwark against the tempests ahead.

But how might we breathe life into such an ambitious vision? The journey begins with the allocation of funds, a substantial financial commitment from both public and private sectors. Government policies must prioritize healthcare spending, incentivizing the modernization of old hospitals and the construction of new ones, equipped for the trials of the future.

Imagine, if you will, medical centers with adaptable spaces, where wards can expand or contract as the tide of patient numbers ebbs and flows. Envision, too, stockpiles of critical supplies managed by sophisticated predictive analytics, ensuring that the right equipment is at hand when seconds count. The adoption of telehealth services should be accelerated, granting remote access to medical care, and reducing the strain on physical facilities.

The implementation of our plan necessitates a phased approach. The initial phase would involve a comprehensive audit of existing healthcare infrastructure, identifying weaknesses and opportunities for improvement. Following this, a strategic framework, tailored to the unique needs of each region, would be developed. Collaboration with architects, engineers, and healthcare professionals will ensure that the facilities designed are not only functional but also healing environments that promote patient recovery and staff well-being.

But what evidence do we have to suggest that such investments yield dividends? Look to the case studies of nations that weathered the pandemic more effectively, where investments in healthcare infrastructure correlated with better outcomes. Consider, too, the economic benefits of a robust healthcare system—a safeguard against the losses incurred by a health crisis.

While our focus remains on bolstering healthcare facilities, let us not overlook alternative solutions. The enhancement of community-based healthcare programs, the integration of artificial intelligence in diagnostics and patient care, and the fortification of global health networks are all worthy pursuits that complement our primary objectives.

Are there risks? Certainly. The misallocation of resources, bureaucratic inertia, and short-sighted policymaking could derail our efforts.

Yet the greater risk lies in inaction. Can we afford to gamble with the future when the stakes are so high?

In summary, the investment in healthcare infrastructure is more than a fiscal endeavor; it's a moral imperative. It is the embodiment of our commitment to the health and security of future generations. With each step forward, we lay the groundwork for a resilient healthcare system capable of withstanding whatever challenges may arise.

The path is laid out before us, a path of foresight and determination. It is a call to build, to innovate, and to safeguard. It is a call we must heed with urgency. For in the aftermath of the COVID-19 pandemic, one truth remains indisputable: the health of our people is the bedrock upon which our society is built, and it is incumbent upon us to fortify that foundation for the ages.

Educational Reforms in Medical Training

In the wake of a global health crisis that tested the mettle of our medical institutions, a new dawn emerges for medical education. The COVID-19 pandemic, like a relentless instructor, imparted lessons that reshaped the landscape of healthcare and the training of its future guardians. As we navigate through the aftermath, we are compelled to examine how these teachings will transform the very essence of medical training.

At the heart of this transformation lies a compelling proposition: to weave the experiences and lessons of COVID-19 into the fabric of medical education, ensuring that the next generation of healthcare professionals is better equipped to handle similar challenges in the future. This is not merely an academic exercise but a vital blueprint for fortifying our healthcare workforce against the unforeseen trials of tomorrow.

The first thread of evidence supporting this claim comes from the exigent shift to virtual learning environments precipitated by the pandemic. Medical schools around the globe, once bastions of traditional, in-person didactics, were compelled to adopt online platforms for education. This pivot revealed both the potential and pitfalls of remote learning. On one hand, students accessed a wealth of digital resources and connected with experts from afar. On the other hand, the lack of hands-on experience and the nuances of patient interaction became glaring deficiencies.

Delving deeper, we observe that this forced adaptation sparked innovation in simulation-based learning. Virtual reality (VR) and augmented reality (AR) technologies began bridging the gap, offering immersive experiences that closely mimic real-life medical scenarios. These tools, once considered supplementary, are now viewed as essential components of a comprehensive medical curriculum. Studies underscore the efficacy of simulation in enhancing clinical skills, with students reporting greater confidence and competence in procedures before encountering actual patients.

Yet, formidable counterarguments arise, questioning the reliance on technology. Critics argue that such tools may never fully replicate the intricacies of human interaction or replace the instinctive learning that occurs in clinical settings. Furthermore, they point to the digital divide, accentuating inequalities in access to technology among students from different socio-economic backgrounds.

In rebuttal, the emphasis lies on the judicious integration of technology with traditional pedagogies. It is not a question of replacement, but rather of enhancement. The pandemic has shown that flexibility in learning methodologies is paramount. Medical training programs must now ensure equitable access to digital resources, fostering an environment where technology acts as a bridge rather than a barrier.

Beyond the realm of digital education, the pandemic has underscored the need for curricula to emphasize public health, health policy, and systems-based practice. Additional evidence of this necessity is found in the surge of medical students volunteering in public health initiatives during the crisis. This experiential learning grounded in real-world challenges has sparked a call for a greater focus on societal health needs within medical training.

The conclusion, reinforced by the weight of these assertions, is inescapable: the evolution of medical education post-COVID is not merely advisable but imperative. We must infuse our curriculum with the acumen gleaned from the pandemic, cultivating a workforce that is technologically adept, versatile in the face of adversity, and deeply attuned to the public health landscape.

So, what does the future hold for the medical trainee? Picture a world where medical students navigate complex clinical simulations with ease, where global health education is not just an elective but a cornerstone of medical training, and where the line between technology and hands-on learning is artfully blurred to produce the most competent and compassionate physicians.

This vision is not a distant dream but a tangible reality within our grasp. With each step toward this new paradigm, we honor the sacrifices made during the pandemic and pay homage to the indomitable spirit of the healthcare community. As we set forth on this path of enlightenment and reform, let our conviction be as steadfast as the purpose that guides us: to emerge from the crucible of COVID-19 with a medical education system that is not only resilient but revolutionary.

Made in the USA
Columbia, SC
08 November 2024

87f9d55b-4c4c-44c3-a04b-f13eb2d3d841R01